LOSE TO WIN

A Cardiologist's Guide to Weight Loss
and
Nutritional Healing

Stephen T. Sinatra, M.D.

Permissions Department
The Lincoln-Bradley Publishing Group
305 Madison Avenue - Suite 1166
New York, NY 10165

Publisher's Cataloging in Publication
(Prepared by Quality Books, Inc.)

Sinatra, Stephen T.
    Lose to win : a cardiologist's guide to weight loss
and nutritional healing / Stephen T. Sinatra.

    p. cm.
    Includes bibliographical references and index.
    ISBN 1-879111-26-8

    1. Medicine, Preventive. 2. Health. 3. Nutrition. 4. Stress
(Psychology)   I. Title
    RA427.8.S5 1992   613
                                    QBI92-508

Printed on approved acid-free paper

Book Design by Electronic Publishing Services, Inc.

1 2 3 4 5 6 7 8 9 10

PREFACE

In the September 16, 1991, MacNeil-Lehrer Report, a provocative discussion regarding the health of the nation was presented by Judy Woodward interviewing a panel of experts. Simply stated, they concluded that cancer and heart disease can be combated by nutritional awareness. *Lose to Win: A Cardiologist's Guide to Weight Loss and Nutritional Healing* is testimony to this insightful premise.

Almost 800 years earlier, in his essays on health, Maimonides, a Mid-Eastern physician, gave a similar prescription for the preservation of health and youth.

THE PRESERVATION OF YOUTH, MAIMONIDES, 1198

Avoid Oversatiety and Fatigue

Exercise Fights Illness

Fat in Meat is Bad

Avoid Milk Products

Wheat is Good for Bread

Music Distracts the Mind and Strengthens the Vital Powers

Emotional Experiences Cause Marked Changes in the Body

Meditation Decreases Evil Thoughts, Sadness and Woes

DEDICATION

For my deceased father, Salvatore Charles Sinatra, who not only taught me how to cook and dance, but also gave me the gift of unconditional love.

ACKNOWLEDGEMENTS

This book could not have been done without the assistance of two creative and powerful colleagues, Julia Molino and Ellen Lieberman. A special thank you goes to Julia Molino, a New York City freelance writer who helped me organize the text. Through her hardworking nature and excellent editorial skills, she kept me focused on ideas that required considerable thought and scrutiny. She always chose the most challenging route, or what I've come to call "taking the high road." I appreciate her persistence in the pursuit of quality.

Ellen Lieberman is a body-oriented therapist and emotional healer from Fairfield, Connecticut. She collaborated with me on two chapters concerning the psychological and emotional struggles associated with weight loss. Her understanding of feminine issues, particularly sexuality, was invaluable. I needed direction that only a woman could provide regarding the basic themes of food, weight, and sexuality. In my experience, I would rank Ellen with the best I have met specializing in these areas.

I also wish to express my heart-felt appreciation to all my office staff who worked incessantly on this project. Grateful thanks go to Jo-Anne Piazza, Rosemary Pontillo, Carol Gustamachio, and Susan Graham. Indeed, my greatest appreciation goes to Peggy Johnson and Patricia Marolt for their enduring efforts in the preparation of this manuscript.

Dr. Bruce Sobin, an internist, was a great help to me, and I appreciated his thoughtful comments and editorialization of the entire text. Dr. Brendan Montano, an internist and expert in depression and weight management, offered some insightful comments. Jan DeMarco, RN, was particularly helpful in making subtle changes in the text. Steve Williford, my editor of Lincoln-Bradley, was especially important in making the book more readable. I appreciated his calming influence and professional direction. I wish to thank Linda and Walter Moore of Memphis, Tennessee, for their hospitality, integrity, and overall guidance.

There are many other individuals who contributed to the work, particularly my patients and clients whom I interviewed. I also wish to acknowledge the men and women who participated in our hospital-based weight-loss program. Their sharing and caring with mutual support for one another not only yielded vital information on the subject of weight loss, but also touched my heart on many occasions.

TABLE OF CONTENTS

INTRODUCTION

My interest in nutrition has been a slow and tedious process. Although being a physician and especially a cardiologist has helped me study the dangers of increased salt and increased saturated fat and cholesterol, I had very little time available to inquire about natural nutritional healing, the perils of vitamin and mineral deficiency, the impact of "polluted water," and the health hazards of heavy metal toxicity in our environment. As a young physician I really had very little understanding of nutrition. It was never emphasized in medical school nor in my internship nor medical residency. My time was consumed in the struggles of health and illness.

As a young physician, I had very little time for understanding why people became sick. As preventive medicine was simply not taught, I focused more on comforting the sick as opposed to prevention. Pharmacological agents became my first line of treatment. After all, the medical profession became drug oriented after the discovery of Penicillin. My training emphasized disease models and interaction with a multitude of pharmacological agents.

For example, high blood pressure or hypertension has been with us for years. In medical school over twenty years ago, the first line of treatment against such high blood pressure was a low-salt diet and weight reduction. Now, however, physicians frequently rely on pharmacological agents as their first choice of treatment. While some still recommend weight loss and a prudent diet, many patients are resistant to this type of therapy. Most people want a simple pill to alleviate the problem. Currently, there are approximately sixty drugs on the market for hypertension alone. Although some of these agents belong to similar classes, the actions are different. Therefore, the emphasis of most cardiologists' time is on pharmacological inquiry.

Trying to determine what drugs will work is a physician's nightmare, much less weighing the potential benefits and hazards of these drugs. So, whatever happened to prevention? Fortunately there is a current shift in the medical community's orientation to illness. Many physicians like myself are now becoming interested in the philosophy and psychology of healing. For example, what is it that makes some people sick while others almost never get ill? Why, for example, does one person catch the flu in a crowd and another doesn't? What is it about certain constitutional weaknesses of individuals that makes them more vulnerable to events?

As a cardiologist, I applied this question to the phenomenon of sudden death. This unexpected event occurs in some clinical studies up to 40 percent of the time as the first symptom of heart disease! This is an awesome statistic for a cardiologist to deal with. As I gained more experience about heart disease, it became increasingly clear to me that heart disease is a process that develops over time. Although heart disease may present suddenly as in the phenomenon of sudden death or heart attack, the process may actually take many years to build.

Contemporary cardiologists are often asked the question, "Why me?" or "Why did I get this illness?" Coronary heart disease is a pathological condition that is really a mosaic of many variables. There are controllable and uncontrollable risk factors. The uncontrollable risk factors include family history, male gender, and advancing age. The controllable risk factors, such as high blood pressure, cigarette smoking, high cholesterol, sedentary living, obesity, and psychological stress are those that enhance the coronary artery disease process, and these risk factors also have a behavioral component. In fact, many of the risk factors are actually an extension of our personalities and character.

For example, high blood pressure may be related to repressed feeling, particularly anger. It became increasingly clear to me over the years that illness has strong emotional and psychological components. For these reasons I have studied psychotherapy and emotional healing over the last 12 years. After studying the impact of personality on illness, I began to publish some of my work in the medical literature. I also held workshops on the psychology of healing and stress and illness. This led me into writing a book entitled *Heartbreak and Heart Disease.* Just as psychological stress affects the heart, metabolic stress can be an equally disturbing factor for not only the heart, but also the general health of the organism.

Similarly, obesity is often related to the emotions. Obesity is in fact the most common metabolic disturbance in humans. Why? Obesity often has it roots in emotional issues, and it is a physical condition that easily manifests itself. When we are overweight, it is difficult to hide from our loved ones, the workplace, or the physician for that matter. Many of my clients, for example, have been evaluated for heart disease as their excessive weight helps to enhance their risk factor profile. There is a growing body of evidence showing that the excess energy stored in fat has adverse implications to health and longevity.

In a study appearing in the medical literature by the Metropolitan Life Insurance Company entitled "Girth and Death," obesity is indeed associated with diastolic hypertension, hypercholesterolemia, and non-insulin dependent diabetes as well as certain cancers. In adults, obesity has been shown to be associated with an increased mortality, particularly cardiovascular disorders.

As a cardiologist, I have had extensive experience and training in the health hazards of obesity and in particular the study of fat, fiber, and cholesterol. I was indeed fortunate to have this training and have incorporated this awareness into my own lifestyle. Awareness can certainly be curative. When it comes down to making food choices, however, many of us are confused and ambivalent. Finding the answers about nutrition and proper eating can be a struggle, particularly for the over-weight individual.

As the former assistant director of a weight loss program at Manchester Memorial Hospital, I had the opportunity to work with many obese individuals on a long-term basis. In this program, the overweight individuals fasted on liquids for several weeks and then were gradually placed on a prudent diet. Coarse carbohydrates, fruits, and vegetables were gradually added as well as meats and low-fat dairy products. The program included behavior modification training and also exercise instructions. As a therapist for a group of 21 participants, I became clearly aware that weight loss is not just a physical struggle. Eating disorders are critically linked to the emotions, focusing on self-esteem, love and acceptance, and even sexuality. I was fortunate to be the leader of a courageous group of men and women. They taught me a lot. We spent six months together for three-hour sessions on a weekly basis.

During this time, I published a study with colleagues on the effects of various types of exercise on both psychological and physical well-being. In this study, we used several groups of women, some who exercised passively (toning tables) and some actively. In one group, we used a low-fat/high-fiber dietary regimen while the others ate a "typical American" diet of processed foods, meats and dairy products. Our study revealed that exercise combined with a low-fat/high-fiber diet had the best results in weight loss with the most improved cholesterol and lipid profile.

This particular study also showed the impact of emotional interaction and support in losing weight. The social facilitation provided by group participation allowed for the greatest support and, therefore, more committed involvement. The group dynamic actually facilitated each individual to lose weight. Thus, by evolution I became surprised with the connection between the psychological and the physical not only in illness but also in wellness.

The study of wellness and preventive medicine, including the impact of psychological and emotional stress, nutritional awareness, participation in exercise, and modification of lifestyle habits, has become the focus of my energies and interests. Although treating illness is still an important factor in my work as a cardiologist, the *challenge of wellness* is always lingering in the background of my thoughts. I feel preventive medicine is really the challenge in contemporary medicine.

Approximately five years ago when I designed our exercise study, I met Roger Buffaloe, an extremely obese individual who had lost 200 pounds of weight. Not only did he lose the weight but he has kept it off for 11 years. He is truly a success story. Over the last few years I had very little communication with Roger until he called me during the summer of 1990, when he asked me to support his diet concept of high-fiber and low-fat meals, which I already believed in. But he actually wanted me to endorse a high-fiber/low-fat product that he had developed, a cookie/cake-like product called *Buffaloe Cookies.*

To say the least, my skepticism was high. How could a cookie or a cake be healthy? And what was so special about this particular product? He asked me to try some of his samples, which I did. I ate the cookies and offered them to several personnel in my office, advising them to eat one cookie with sixteen ounces of water as a replacement for breakfast and/or lunch. Everyone liked the taste and the variety and some lost weight. I even gave them to my mother, one of my best critics, and she too liked them, calling them the "Roger Rabbit Cakes." (I tried telling her that it was Buffaloe, not Rabbit, but she didn't get it.) I began to take the product seriously and over the course of four weeks, I lost five pounds while my cholesterol dropped 22 points. I was excited. I called Roger and told him that I would support him in his efforts.

While returning from California where I had just endorsed the Roger Buffaloe high-fiber/low-fat cookie, an idea came to me at approximately 35,000 feet. I had the insight, or perhaps it was a fantasy, that healthy food would become not only a major focus in the 1990's, but also the cardinal ingredient in preventive medicine. While flying above the clouds, I began to think of Roger Buffaloe's high-fiber/low-fat cookies. What if other products could be devised with a high-fiber/low-fat profile that tasted equally as good? Could a high-fiber/low-fat concept actually make a difference in the health care of this country? Could it help lower the incidence of coronary heart disease?

Like a beanstalk, my fantasy grew and grew and soon became real. With a group of interested physicians, I opened a "healthy" food store called *Natural Rhythms,* in Manchester, Connecticut. I personally screened all the products for low-fat and high-fiber content. In order to get the *Natural Rhythms* seal of approval, manufacturers would have to make products with less than 20 percent fat, keeping sugar, salt, and cholesterol to a minimum. I learned very quickly that many health food products were not really healthy at all. For example, one of the best organic granolas advertised in the country was preserved with tropical coconut oil, which is extremely dangerous to the health of the heart. Banana chips, I found, were actually deep fried in similar tropical oils.

It became clear to me that buying "health food" required active scrutiny. I began to read incessantly about fat, fiber, vitamins, chemical pollutants, and the healing aspects of nutrition. *Natural Rhythms* became the doctor's health food store. I requested organic produce, grains, pastas and juices, and actually began to recommend sea vegetables to my clients, as well as vitamins and minerals. I was learning new things at an alarming rate. I began to do computer searches in the medical literature, for example, and was shocked to find that 178 articles were written on vitamins alone in the last six months which were germane to the internist and family practitioner and of course their patients. Such culmination of my energies has become the focus of *Lose to Win: A Cardiologist's Guide to Weight-Loss and Nutritional Healing.*

This book is not about dieting and deprivation, but rather focuses on nurturing the body with nutritional and emotional healing. Many of my patients now ask, "What can I eat?" This book provides simple answers: *Low-fat/high-fiber foods.* I employ the metaphor of "the good, the bad, and the issue" in an analysis of fiber, cholesterol, and fat. I show *vitamins* and minerals as antagonists to a multitude of chemical pollutants. You will investigate the "nuts and bolts" of nutrition—the *real* reasons behind obesity and why we cannot lose weight. The weight is on the surface, manifesting itself in "body armor," but being overweight is just another way that the body sends a signal to the psyche for the need to heal itself.

The *emotional issues* of obesity are indeed deep and buried in the personality. Some portions of the text will elicit an emotional response from you: hope, inspiration, sadness, fear, or anger. The content may actually challenge you to see where the core of your weight problem is.

Lose to Win is about giving up the struggle with dieting and having fun. It focuses on a *lifestyle* that facilitates nutritional awareness but not starvation. This book is not merely a self-help manual; it is really about expanding one's consciousness. The 1990's are a time of awareness, of taking responsibility for oneself, and living in harmony with one's body. *Lose to Win* supports a weight-reduction process in which the individual opens doors to creativity and aliveness. This book is not so much about becoming thin, but about making a real goal that is larger than weight loss. It is about getting in touch with your true self.

Lose to Win is available at special quantity discounts.

For details regarding quantity purchases, write or telephone:

Special Markets
The Lincoln-Bradley Publishing Group
305 Madison Avenue - Suite 1166
New York, NY 10165
(212) 953-1125

CHAPTER 1

DIETS DON'T WORK:
THE ROGER BUFFALOE STORY

Roger Buffaloe was a man who while only in his mid-thirties weighed nearly 400 pounds. Roger Buffaloe is now a man who weighs 186 pounds, as he has for the past 11 years. How did he come to weigh so much and how is it that after years of dieting (and failing) he finally lost over 200 pounds? What caused Roger to become obese and why couldn't he stop eating excessively? Roger is an example of one of the many overweight people in our society who are morbidly obese (40 percent or more above desirable weight). Four out of every 10 Americans are overweight (20% or more above desired weight), and one out of five, or 34 million adults, is obese. Why?

There has been much discussion about this among the medical community. Books have been written on the psychological, the behavioral, and the systemic causes of obesity. I can't say there is not a comprehensive program that addresses all of these concerns – there are many. You may have tried some of them. But if they haven't worked for you in the past, read on.

Let's review the contributing factors to overeating so we all can have an understanding of the basis of eating disorders and begin at the same point. First of all, *stop feeling guilty*. Regardless of whether you are 10 pounds or 200 pounds overweight, don't beat yourself up saying, "I shouldn't have; I must stop myself; I must have control; I must deny myself pleasure in the short term in order to gain long-term results."

RULE NUMBER ONE: DENIAL OF PLEASURE CAN LEAD TO OBESITY AND EARLY DEATH

Well, you might say, I can understand how eating disorders can lead to early death, but how can denial of pleasure? As a cardiologist and psychotherapist, it is easy for me to see that self-denial can cause extreme unhappiness that sets up stress and heartbreak that lead to heart disease and frequently death. *Denial of love, denial of human contact, and denial of emotional outlets clog the system just as surely as do fats and cholesterol!*

Always doing what we "think" is best and not acting on what we truly feel, stopping ourselves from doing what we always wanted because of fear of rejection or loss, or denying ourselves the simple sensual pleasures of life that came so easily in childhood stops the natural flow of energy that we depend on as our very lifeforce. Lying in a field of wild grass or in a pile of freshly raked leaves, watching the clouds drift by and finding fantasy in reality, or smelling the aroma of hot cookies being taken from the oven and the joy of allowing the moist dough to melt on the tongue - these are the things that as adults we forbid ourselves. Why? Because we are busy, because we must efficiently rake the leaves, not scatter them, because we are overweight and must not eat a sweet cookie. But don't we still long for the feeling of crisp leaves or freshly mowed grass next to our skin? Don't we still want the cookie?

In most cases, yes, we do. And one of two things usually happens: (1) We deny ourselves and through a series of similar victories and perhaps one or two slip ups, we lose weight. Great! But denial of pleasure breeds resentment and resentment harbors contempt, fostering feelings of guilt and frustration. (2) Because our approach to food was seen as friend or enemy, we give up in defeat, vowing to start anew tomorrow, or we binge and cry that we might as well be fat and fulfilled. Wrong. We might be full, but we are not fulfilled. We are guilty and self-loathing, and these unforgiving feelings start the cycle of denial all over again.

This is what happened to Roger Buffaloe and at nearly 400 pounds, how could he possibly recommend anything but absolute denial? Because he learned through trial and error that complete denial leads to complete failure. We must allow ourselves foods that we enjoy but in a manner that is contained. Less can be more. I suggest *awareness* over denial. As Roger now realizes, if he eats a piece of bread without butter, he can have more bread than if he eats it with butter. This is awareness. This is choice. And it's not deprivation. He can still eat bread, preferably a high-fiber, textured, whole-grain variety that will give him a satisfied, full feeling without doing damage to the body.

The other night, for example, my friends and I had a celebratory dinner that was entirely low-fat, yet as delicious as any Thanksgiving dinner I've had. The menu consisted of roasted turkey, fresh green and yellow beans, a pasta salad, and a salad of cucumbers and tomatoes, as well as bread. We ended the meal with fresh fruit pies. Because the rest of the meal was low-fat, I chose not to deprive myself and to have a small piece of pie, though I realized that the crust of the pie was made with lard, a pure animal fat frequently used in baking. A three-inch piece of pie contains 15-20 grams of fat, which was more than the entire meal I just consumed. The American Heart Association recommends a daily diet of no more than 65 grams of fat a day for an average sized man such as myself. Since the meal contained minimal fat, I was able not to deprive myself, with the awareness that the total fat content for this meal, including the "forbidden" pie, was only about 30 grams! This is eating with awareness. This is curative.

A typical fast food meal, on the other hand, including a double cheeseburger, french fries, a shake, and an apple pie, contains an alarming 70-80 grams of fat! And this is only one meal. If this lifestyle were continued, one could conceivably eat 200-225 grams of fat a day! This is not only "fattening," but dangerous! What, however, if you can't stop with just one bite of bread with butter or with one cookie?

RULE NUMBER TWO: FORGIVE YOURSELF

If we allow ourselves a little bit of what we are being denied, in a program of awareness we can become masters of our own enjoyment and be fulfilled (More on this later as we get into "how." For now, let's stick with "why."). And if we are unable to stay within the contained means and do indeed overeat, and we continue to berate ourselves, it only adds to feelings of failure and self-doubt. On the other hand, if we can allow some leeway for human frailty we can begin anew.

Let's not kid ourselves, though. Eating our favorite foods in a contained environment isn't always easy. A taste of ice cream may lead to an entire bowl. But rather than requiring willpower or discipline, Roger found the key was forgiving himself and getting support from others.Roger was and is extremely disciplined in many ways. He overcame a learning disability to teach himself how to read after quitting high school because he was labeled "fat and stupid." Having managed a business at only 16 years old and turning it from a Mom and Pop shop into a very profitable venture, he received his high school equivalency degree and later became a highly successful businessman. Roger never lacked willpower. But he did lack support. His teachers thought he was dumb and lazy. His father criticized him for making poor grades and his mother just didn't understand what could be the problem with his weight and lack of control over his appetite.

Frequently, overweight adults result from families where achieving was more important than being and where there was little acceptance of the children as they really were because they were not as the parents wanted them to be. Does this mean we should blame our parents for not giving us unconditional love? Not necessarily. They probably received similar treatment from their parents, or from a society that encouraged them to believe this is the way to instill success into their children. On the contrary, too much pressure (for adults, much less children), only tempts us to rebel or to loath our shortcomings – what we have come to call failure – just as eating one cookie is a failure that may lead to the hopelessness of eating ten.

RULE NUMBER THREE: GET SUPPORT

On top of trying to lose weight, we have work pressures, family pressures, and if overweight, may very well have sexual issues begging to be resolved. Were does one "problem" stop and the other begin? We have a bad day at work and so follow it up with a cocktail or two. Our libidos get activated and, rather than risk rejection, or worse yet, nudity, we try satisfying it with creamy ice cream. Of course, the cycle goes on and on. In an *aware* consciousness, however, we can direct our energies. We can call or meet with others who know our struggles and who can encourage us to come over for a glass of juice instead of a cocktail, or who can talk us through our work frustrations and then help us to plan dinner. With this type of understanding, planning social occasions and meals can truly be rewarding rather than dreaded.

As Roger neared the 400 pound mark, he lost more and more friends. Not because they thought Roger was any less interesting or amusing than he was before, but because *Roger* felt too vulnerable to accept their invitations. He became more and more isolated, even from his wife, literally barricading himself with fat and cutting off the very support that is so helpful in achieving any goal. Just as Roger was carrying nearly 400 pounds of physical weight, he also had approximately 400 pounds of emotional burden. His psychic pain was devastating – he thought of himself as an outcast and acted it, becoming lonely and alone. How many of us, when in pain, turn away from those who love us, those who could help us most? And as friends, how many of us refuse to support another in a similar situation? What is not needed is, "Are you eating again? You are just going to get fatter and fatter." But rather, "Instead of eating that bag of potato chips, can I fix you a crunchy bowl of popcorn?"

RULE NUMBER FOUR: EAT HIGH–FIBER AND LOW–FAT FOODS

One of the things Roger learned with his dieting is that texture is frequently as satisfying as flavor. When craving ice cream, the creaminess of a low-fat frozen yogurt can usually fulfill the urge. And now there are new products on the market that allow the taste of ice cream without the fat or sugar. While I personally prefer and recommend food in its most natural form, recent food engineering has made possible tasty "diet" foods. The creation of Nutrasweet, the sugar substitute, and Simplesse, the fat substitute, for example, have enabled people who are resistant to natural-food eating to be able to watch their fat and sugar intake while still enjoying the foods they like. Remember, however, that these food substitutes are not natural ingredients and while they may have been approved by the FDA as being non-harmful, they are not a natural approach to weight loss, which is what this book encourages. This is why I suggest having a small portion of ice cream or an entire cup of yogurt to stop a craving for a creamy comfort food. But ultimately, you know what type of eater you are and what you are willing and unwilling to try. I am writing this book, however, to encourage you at least to try this approach: *Awareness over denial.*

High-fiber and low-fat choices will allow you to lose weight without giving up naturally good-tasting food. This has been substantiated by many of my patients. They started out taking my dietary recommendations for a high-fiber/low-fat diet in order to heal their hearts. A diet low in saturated fats reduces the level of "bad" cholesterol that contributes to hardening of the arteries and heart attacks. A diet high in fiber keeps the body and appetite nourished while allowing most of the refuse of the digested food to be flushed away by the intestines. While my patients started on this diet to heal their hearts, they ended up losing weight! This is why *pasta is now considered a healthy food for dieters,* especially if it is a *pasta made from whole-wheat or semolina flour,* as we now know these are complex carbohydrates. Since they are not made with refined sugars, any increases in blood sugar that occur after eating is gradual and healthy. Add a simple sauce of vegetables, for which I give many recipes later, and this is a perfect "diet" meal. Of course, we must return to the idea of eating with *awareness.* One plate of pasta will more often leave us feeling full and "rewarded" than two or three plates of large curd cottage cheese – a typical "diet" food – and with fewer calories!

When Roger was losing weight, many of the newly engineered diet foods were unavailable, but this is not what caused him to turn to a high-fiber/low-fat diet. He tried every diet available: The Scarsdale Diet, The Grapefruit Diet, The Aviator's Diet, and protein drinks. With none of them, however, could he keep the weight off when he returned to "normal" eating. Obviously it was the "normal" eating that needed to be changed. Eleven years ago the public was just learning about the benefits of fiber, and Roger took it to heart. He would carry with him pure fiber crackers that even he says did not have a good taste, which he would snack on when needed. And he would eat fruit, a source of natural sugar, when he felt his energy was low. Being a steak lover, Roger didn't eliminate red meat from his diet, but he did cut it back significantly, and he would always remove all the visible fat before taking even one bite. In this way he didn't feel deprived, yet his eating was *contained.* He was aware that if he ate the steak, he could not follow it with bread, butter, and salty french fries.

RULE NUMBER FIVE: AVOID SALT, SUGAR, AND CAFFEINE WHILE CONSUMING AS MUCH WATER AS POSSIBLE

Now this may sound like denial, but let me explain. Salt, sugar, and caffeine do not need to be avoided altogether, but they should be used in moderation for both improved health and weight loss. You see, there is a direct relationship between caffeine intake and sugar cravings. It works like this: Sugar intake quickly boosts the blood sugar and just as quickly lowers it, thereby causing a sugar craving in order to boost energy again. Caffeine works in a similar manner: It boosts our energy level and drops again, thus causing a craving for a sweet or another cup of coffee to keep us going. While increasing sugar consumption increases energy and staves off hunger pangs induced by the dropping of blood sugar from a previous sweet or cup of coffee, it creates a cycle of eating sugar and/or drinking coffee as often as every two hours! Such increased sugar intake can obviously lead to an increase in accumulated fat.

The way to prevent or even to stop this cycle, is to begin your day with a complex carbohydrate that will slowly be converted to blood sugar. Instead of the quick boost that a sweet roll gives, a bowl of oatmeal, for example, will allow a more gradual increase and subsequent decrease in blood sugar and, therefore, will prolong the time of satiety. Eating a complex carbohydrate that also has high amounts of fiber, such as shredded wheat or a *Buffaloe Cookie*, will control hunger even longer because fiber taken with water or another liquid will bulk in the gastrointestinal tract, thus creating a feeling of fullness.

If you choose a high fiber, complex carbohydrate for breakfast, you may safely have a cup of coffee (without added sugar) without beginning the sugar/caffeine cycle. While the caffeine may cause a food craving, it will be satisfied by the gradual release of energy caused by the slow burning of the complex carbohydrate as opposed to the need of a quick fix with a processed sugar item. Remember, anything that is sugary tasting or sticky feeling is probably made with processed sugar, such as the table sugar found in commercially packaged breads and cereals; so *read labels!* The ingredients are listed in order of the highest quantities of ingredients. Therefore, if sugar is the first or second ingredient, it may comprise the majority of the product.

Breakfast may begin or prevent a day of overeating, so choose wisely. Following on the left are some foods to try to replace the foods listed on the right:

AVOID	REPLACE WITH
Sugared cereals	Whole grain cereals, oatmeal
White bread	Wholewheat bread
Commercial pancakes with processed syrup	Buckwheat cakes with honey

(cont'd)	**AVOID**	**REPLACE WITH**
	Belgian waffles	Whole grain waffles
	with whipped cream	with spreadable fruit
	Sweet rolls	Rolled oats
	Blueberry muffins	Bran muffins
	Cookies	Roger Buffaloe Cakes or
		Cookies

When making food choices, invoke the general rule of thumb that is easy to remember: **THE CLOSER THE FOOD IS TO ITS NATURAL ORIGINAL FORM, THE BETTER.** In other words, whenever possible, buy wholewheat bread from your local baker instead of white bread from the grocery market. While you can still use "convenience foods," choose frozen waffles from a health food store instead of packed toaster cakes. You can make a batch of buckwheat pancakes by merely adding water to a mix available at many of the farm stores that sell fresh produce instead of using a processed biscuit or pancake mix.

Even my 11 year old son prefers multigrain pancakes (my recipe follows in the *Recipes For Life* section) to those he gets in his friends' homes, because my pancakes have a chewier texture and a fuller flavor. And I serve them to him with pure maple syrup tapped from the trees around a cabin I have in Vermont. Okay, okay, you don't have to tap your own trees, but if you can splurge for a jug of pure maple syrup instead of the commercially packaged brands, not only will the flavor be more robust, but it will be healthier as well. Another healthy choice is to spread a layer of honey on the pancakes. While dousing them in either syrup or honey is not advised, a small amount gives flavor and satisfaction.

I also recommend the consumption of generous quantities of fluids at breakfast, whether in juice, decaffeinated beverage, vitamins, or even just plain water – a cardinal ingredient in health. Water consumption cleanses the organs of excess sodium that is often hidden in many of today's foods, especially commercially packaged convenience foods such as canned soups, boxed mixes and sauces, and even sweets. *Selected foods especially high in sodium include pickles, ketchup, mustard, soy sauce, and pickled fish,* to mention a few. *Sodas* can be one of the worst offenders of a low sodium diet. Even some low calorie carbonated soft drinks have sodium in them. So if you are in the habit of drinking a diet beverage instead of water with a meal or to quench thirst, it will not only prevent a good opportunity to cleanse the system, but will also add to its contamination.

Remember that high sodium intake also contributes to high blood pressure and heart disease, so *it's wise to replace all sodas with water,* tap or bottled, and to drink as much water as possible throughout the day. In addition to sodium and sugar content, *many soft drinks contain emulsifiers, artificial coloring, phosphoric acid, and antifoaming agents.* These chemicals cause metabolic stress to our bodies, as do other additives, preservatives, and synthetic agents commonly used in processed foods – setting up our next rule: Read Labels and Eat Natural.

RULE NUMBER SIX: READ LABELS AND EAT NATURAL

Controversies regarding nutrition seem to be on the news almost nightly. For example, *60 Minutes* recently ran a program regarding the pros and cons of new proposals for food labeling. Consumers in the past who have relied heavily on food labels for nutritional information have now been rescued by the FDA with their recent policies for clearing up misleading advertising information. They are tackling such dilemmas as how much fat is low-fat? What does low-sodium mean? Or for that matter, what does low-calorie mean? Manufacturers in the past have boasted that a product can be "cholesterol-free," yet it may contain large amounts of saturated fat which is eventually *turned* into cholesterol in the body. With the new definition, cholesterol-free will be legally defined as less than two milligrams of cholesterol per serving. Likewise, "low cholesterol" will be less than 20 mg of cholesterol. "High-fiber" is another term that is frequently unregulated, but the new legislation will require specific grams of fiber per serving. New FDA standardizations will make it easier for consumers to rely on factual nutritional information. Not only will consumers be able to determine the amount of calories in a particular item, they will also be given information about the number of calories from fat, the amount of saturated fatty acids (SFAs), cholesterol, fiber, carbohydrate, protein, sodium, potassium, and even information regarding vitamins and minerals.

Okay. Enough about the good news. What's happening with the bad news? What are the Feds doing about the chemicals, preservatives and other harmful ingredients that are added to commercially packaged foods? Although the FDA has issued formal regulations on literally hundreds of food additives, these are agents that are still listed as GRAS (Generally Regarded As Safe). These food additives are chemicals used in artificial flavors, colors, bleaches, emulsifiers, softeners, thickeners, hydrogenators, deodorizers, conditioners, antioxidants, fortifiers, driers, alkalizers, firming agents, stabilizers, and buffers. They will add color and eye appeal to food that does not need refrigeration, but for all practical purposes, these agents are literally "dead;" that is, they do nothing useful but extend shelf life. And are they *really* safe?

DON'T BECOME A GARBAGE DUMP!

Two commonly used GRAS additives, butylated hydroxyanisole and butylated hydroxytoluene, frequently referred to as BHA and BHT, are antioxidants made from *petroleum*. BHA and BHT are found in almost every processed food, including cereals, shortening, ice cream, dairy foods, peanut butter, potato chips, meats, dressings, snacks, etc. They do indeed give foods an extended shelf life and also prevent rancidity. However, these additives have been reported as having a casual relationship to allergies and nervous system disorders.

Monosodium glutamate (MSG) is also considered a food enhancer in thousands of foods. "Convenience foods," such as TV dinners, processed meats, tenderizers, and dressings, contain considerable quantities of MSG. In fact, industry officials indicate that MSG is the most widely utilized chemical flavoring agent. Since MSG has been utilized since 1907, it has a long history of use and has been closely scrutinized. It has been proven to show some side effects such as asthma, palpitations, chest pain, weakness, and heartburn that may occur in both children and adults. In experimental animals, MSG has also been shown to cause permanent brain damage. Headache is probably the leading symptom of MSG intake, frequently sending patients to their doctors for unnecessary evaluations and interventions when a good nutritional history and diet change would suffice.

What does this all mean to the consumer? Unfortunately, the average consumer takes in thousands of chemical additives in his food. But we cannot blame it all on the food industry. We really do want convenience, speedy preparations, a longer shelf life, and quick and easy menus. Major food companies take advantage of the consumer by advertising campaigns that are impressive but sometimes misleading. Although processed foods may be inexpensive, the consumer does pay a price in terms of physical symptoms and perhaps increased susceptibility to illness.

We need to become more discriminating shoppers. Read labels and look for ones that say "no preservatives," "free from additives." But do not be seduced by reading "no preservatives;" also look to see if artificial flavorings or colorings have been added. Watch out for the camouflage labels which list "natural flavoring, hydrolyzed protein, sodium caseinate, and autolyzed yeast." These are used frequently to disguise MSG. We need to be suspicious of chemical names and ingredient abbreviations.

Avoid BHA, BHT, sodium nitrate, sodium nitrite, caffeine, sulfur dioxide, butyric acid, dietylene glycol, sodium benzoate, and amyl acetate. If you do not understand the language, or feel you need a Ph.D. or an M.D. degree to figure out the contents, then the product should be avoided. Be aware of the toxic ingredient *aluminum,* and be particularly cognizant of the use of *white flour additives.* Additives such as *ammonium chloride, potassium bromate, and propionic acid* (sodium or calcium propionate) are all unnatural to living organisms. Just as industrial chemicals can pollute the environment, these chemicals, added to breads, pollute the body. We need to realize that additives and chemicals actually add nothing to the nutritional value to foods. They are frequently added to make inferior substances taste better.

But, the far better option is to consider natural and organically grown foods. Try to learn about and seek out organic foods which are free of pesticides and chemical fertilizers. Organic gardening indicates that the soil is free of any artificially produced fertilizers for several years or even decades. Natural foods are gradually becoming more and more popular with consumers. Although the consumer may pay a few pennies more and may have to accept shorter shelf lives, the dividend can be a healthier body and mind. We have to be willing to *give up precooked, instant, refined, and chemically treated foods.* If you want good health, you need to compromise and take more responsibility for the ingredients you put into your body. Go out and be a detective and guard your body since this is the only one you will ever have.

RULE NUMBER SEVEN: MOVE!

The definition of a calorie is a unit for measuring energy. This means that for every calorie that we take in, we must expend an equal amount of energy in order to remain at a balanced weight. When we take in more calories than we expend, we gain weight. When we expend more energy than we take in, we lose weight. And when the two are balanced, we can remain at a constant weight.

Okay, so you know this already. You may even feel hopeless that you could ever expend more energy than you take in because you are not an athletic person. Don't believe it. Any little activity greater than you are doing now will burn more calories. So even if you are consuming the same amount of food today as you were yesterday, but you add a bit more movement to your day, you will lose weight slowly. Now, add to today's diet some foods less dense in calories than yesterday and you are losing weight twice as fast.

Notice that I say, "movement," not exercise. I think exercise can sometimes be a scary word. People visualize running down the road in sweaty shorts and sneakers or pumping iron. Professionally speaking, I must say I don't recommend either. Both put a tremendous amount of stress on the heart muscle and other muscles and tendons that pop and burst because of overzealous or incorrect use. Let's take it easy.

Remember, this is a program of non-denial, or enjoyment.

Let's start out *walking*. The evening breeze is cool and spring or fall crispness might be in the air. Or perhaps there is a beautiful red August moon that you can see from your window. Get up. Walk outdoors. Enjoy nature. This is the holistic way of living. Mind and body are one. Human life and wildlife are on the same planet. Let's enjoy each other as we are all part of the same universe. Even if you can't find time to walk every day (though I think you might, once you get used to the beauty of the landscape), think of every little movement you make and take it one step beyond. Walk out to the driveway to get the mail instead of picking it up in your car on the way home. Walk around the bed to make up the other side rather than reaching over. While watching television, my teenage daughter does leg lifts. Think of this not as strenuous exercise, but as an efficient use of exercise time!

When Roger first started losing weight, he couldn't even reach over to tie his shoes. He couldn't walk more than a few yards. Four hundred pounds is a lot of weight to move around. So he started walking out for the newspaper each morning and taking out the trash. He even began cleaning out closets. Roger was a successful businessman who, if he wanted, could hire a housekeeper to clean closets. But Roger knew that each added movement would add to his successful weight loss. Every little movement counts. Like a savings account, Roger added more and more movement to his daily regimen until he accumulated the lifestyle he has today. Now he plays racquetball three times a week and even won his division in the North Carolina State Championship in 1986. He was one of the oldest men to win this title in the United States – and to think that only six years previously he could barely walk far enough to take the trash out.

RULE NUMBER EIGHT: ADD VITAMINS AND MINERALS TO YOUR DIET

Eating vitamins and minerals will keep your body healthy while it is going through the strenuous shifts and changes that occur with weight loss. Remember that your metabolism is going to change. And if you are replacing high fat and sugary foods in your diet with natural foods, you are going to have some noticeable physical differences. For example, you may have larger bowel movements, but this may remove important minerals as well. While hair and eyes may become shinier, your skin may at first break out and then clear to a creamy complexion. We call this process elimination and purification. The old "garbage" that is in your body is being flushed out and replaced with healthier natural foods. Taking various vitamins and minerals, or foods high in certain of these, will aid in this transition.

Once you are on a balanced diet, you can decide if you want to take supplements or choose to get your vitamins and minerals through your food. I suggest a combination. Being a physician, I have read numerous studies on the benefits of adding high amounts of vitamin C to the diet. For example, I drink 500 mg of a powdered vitamin C a day – and it tastes like orange juice! Some minerals I prefer to get through food. Again, I have read studies on certain foods, such as seaweed or miso that are beneficial in not only warding off disease, but also in healing because of their high mineral content. Now you might not think of eating seaweed, but in a vegetable broth it tastes like the escarole of the traditional Italian Wedding Soup and it is one of the healthiest and most healing foods available. Later in the book I will tell you more about vitamins and minerals and about foods that heal.

When Roger began his high-fiber/low-fat diet, he began reading everything he could about vitamins and minerals. From there he became acquainted with his local health food store and learned about natural eating. He saw the packaged foods that were being sold there. Although much better than the packaged foods available on supermarket shelves, many of the "health food" products contained calories that he felt were needlessly wasted in fats and high-fructose sugars. What he wanted was a food product that would satiate his hunger, keep his taste buds happy, and yet be good for him, supplying him with necessary vitamins and minerals.

Remembering that Roger was a crackerjack businessman, it's not surprising that he became determined to come up with one. Roger admits he was a foodaholic and a workaholic, bordering on alcoholism at times. Perhaps as a carry over from his youth when people misread his learning disability as slowness, he became determined to perform every task to the best of his abilities. This need to "prove himself" most likely contributed to his obesity. The voices of his critical father and disapproving teachers repeated in his head until he became as hard on himself as they were on him. So while he created successful businesses, several grocery markets, night clubs, a restaurant, and a luxury auto dealership, he ate to sublimate his own hidden fears, pain, and anxieties. The more he achieved, the more he ate, and the worse he felt about himself.

NOW THAT'S FAT!

Roger tells the story of the time he and another 400 pound friend got into Roger's Corvette in front of his luxury auto dealership. With much effort, they struggled into the low-slung car and once seated, attempted to shut the doors simultaneously. But neither could. Between them, there was just too much man inside the little car. With his employees watching, Roger didn't want to bear further humiliation by getting out and admitting defeat, so he became determined to get the doors shut. First he leaned outward and told his friend to pull his door shut, then to reverse the action while Roger pulled his shut. Since their first attempts were not successful, their repeated efforts created a rocking motion and the two 400 pound men swayed from side to side as they tried to physically reposition, and figuratively, remold their huge bodies into ones that would fit into a svelte Corvette. As the car rocked from side to side, Roger admits it must have been a funny sight. His employees began gathering at the windows of the dealership and laughing hysterically. Roger waved to them, smiling and encouraging their fun while pushing down his true feelings of hurt and shame. Finally, they got the doors shut and left behind the embarrassing situation.

It was with the same single-minded resolve that Roger finally decided to lose weight. Not long after becoming stuck in the chair of a shoe store and dumping an unsuspecting lady on the floor when he stood up and took a row of connected seats with him, he was rushed to the hospital with an inability to breathe. Roger had been feeling some discomfort sleeping and breathing, he was running a slight temperature, and his head felt stuffed. His doctor examined him, listening to his chest, and could find nothing more. He diagnosed a cold. After almost a month the symptoms got worse, so Roger saw another physician. Again the doctor could not hear congestion in Roger's chest when he listened with a stethoscope. Again, a cold was the diagnosis. Because Roger felt so badly, he was sure there was something more. He asked for a chest x-ray. And when it was returned, the doctor suggested Roger be immediately hospitalized. Roger had a severe case of pneumonia, which couldn't be detected with a stethoscope through the layers of fat around his 60-inch chest.

When Roger was checked into the hospital, they took his vital signs and wanted to check his weight. However, the nurses feared he was too large for even medical scales which went up to only 300 pounds and told him he might have to go to their laundry room to be weighed. His shame and humiliation were intense. Luckily, they brought in a special scale that saved him the further pain of being weighed as cargo. As he was waiting for the process to be over, he saw a cadaver being wheeled out of a room. When Roger learned that the man had died from complications of pneumonia, a "click" went off in his head. Roger had an advanced case of pneumonia resulting from difficulty diagnosing the disease because of his weight. Roger suddenly realized – and believed – that one way or another, his overeating was going to kill him.

As a cardiologist, I see many overweight people who end up as cardiac deaths. Clinical studies show that obese people move less than thinner people and many heart attacks occur within a short time after a high-fat meal. Movement and light low-fat meals are two ways of contributing to a healthy heart. If it hadn't been the pneumonia that scared Roger into the realization that his weight was dangerous, it might have been a heart attack, and he might not have been as lucky. As it was, Roger left the hospital cured of his pneumonia and determined to lose weight. The energy he used in building his businesses and hiding the pain of his fat he now channeled into losing weight. Just as he previously gave his entire attention to work and food, Roger made losing weight his new obsession.

While in the hospital Roger had time to analyze his eating habits. He had been dieting for at least 20 years and nothing had worked, so he deduced that diets don't work. The only "diet" he could count on was the age-old way of eating less and eating lighter. He didn't just worry about counting calories. Instead, he focussed on lowering his fat intake. If he reduced the amount of red meats and oily foods he was consuming, he would need to increase fiber foods in order to eat less and yet feel full. It just made sense.

So Roger set a reasonable goal – one he felt he could achieve – before he had even another taste of butter. Once he achieved his goal, however, he then started to "play games" with his diet. He would allow himself bread without butter except for the last bite, on which he would smear just enough to get the full taste. After a short time, he surprisingly learned that he no longer liked the taste of butter. It was too heavy, too oily, too strong.

Roger lost weight. The people who had known him his whole life didn't recognize him and others whom he didn't know well would say, "I heard you lost weight, but I couldn't imagine this much. How did you do it?" Word spread and he would find more people in his office asking for weight-loss advice than at the checkout counter in his grocery store. He told them about eating low-fat and high-fiber foods, but many of them didn't understand about whole grains and fiber. He was thrilled about his own success in losing weight and wanted to help others. Just as he shed his fat and his fat lifestyle, Roger sold his grocery markets and opened a weight-loss center where he could teach people about fat, fiber, and vitamins. Like Roger, I believe in eating with awareness. The rest of this book will teach you this philosophy.

CHAPTER 2

OBESITY: THE PROBLEM

The United States population is never at a loss to find new ways to lose weight. We all know there is an abundance of diets available. Some are seemingly more successful than others, but any diet will work for a motivated individual. The odds of maintaining weight loss, however, are discouraging. Most diets result in the majority of individuals regaining their weight when they resume "normal" eating patterns. Studies show that only a small fraction of overweight persons who succeed in weight loss are able to keep the weight off for more than a short period of time.

As we saw in the Roger Buffaloe story, "Diets Don't Work." Dieting in general implies a temporary change in the way we eat, instead of a permanent shift in the way we perceive ourselves in our relationship to food. Diet also implies deprivation. When one utilizes deprivation, food is not a friend, but rather an enemy. Typically, it is felt that self-sacrifice is the only way to achieve success, and that enjoyment of food is a sin that leads to an overpowering sense of frustration and failure. This emotional roller coaster can be quite disturbing. An ideal diet comes from one's own consciousness and individualization. Such insight and awareness of what is healthy and what is unhealthy, what you can live with and live without, is really the key to losing weight.

For example, people who starve themselves or force themselves to eat unusual or unpalatable foods are bound to fail in the long run. Clinical studies have demonstrated that people who participate in these diets fail to achieve long-term weight loss and may often end up weighing more. A more practical approach would be to gradually increase and improve the quality of one's diet by eating a variety of healthy low-fat/high-fiber foods that taste good. Just as most people can change from whole milk to two percent milk and eventually lose their taste for whole milk, similar changes may take place with just a little experimentation. We all have food preferences. The secret is to utilize our favorite foods, making adjustments to balance them with less caloric or healthier choices.

For example, one serving of premium ice cream contains two to three times the calories of a serving of frozen yogurt. Therefore, the choice is to eat more frozen yogurt or less ice cream. This awareness is a small but crucial step in *nutritional healing*. A long-term weight loss program, therefore, is really a lifestyle that is palatable and somewhat calorie-deficient, but enjoyable. Over time, the brain makes the gradual switch into believing that frozen yogurt is the same as ice cream.

Calorie is a word that frequently comes up in daily conversations, but not everyone knows its definition. A calorie is a measure of energy. When we speak about food, we give it a number reflecting the amount of energy it yields when it burns. It takes energy to perform activites. If the body needs a steady supply of calories to fuel it with energy, any food supply will do. But if we supply our bodies with an overabundance of energy in the form of calories, this creates weight gain. In simple terms, the problem with being overweight is a problem of energy balance. Energy balance is the relationship between energy intake and energy expenditure. For example, it takes approximately 100 calories of energy to walk one mile. If we walk a mile and then drink a 200 calorie frosted shake, we will not lose weight but only add to it. When the energy balance is positive, the extra calories are stored as fat. When the energy balance is negative, fat is broken down to provide the necessary energy the body needs. This simple fact is a cardinal ingredient in weight loss.

OFF THE COUCH AND MOVE ANYTHING!

Keeping this energetic point of view in mind, we need to ask how the body conserves and expends energy. The body is also utilizing energy at rest as well as during exercise. This is reflected in one's basal metabolic rate (BMR) or the energy required to sustain the basic functions of life (breathing, heart rate, organic functions, etc.). The BMR may vary from one individual to another as well as from one activity to another.

For example, the athlete may have a higher metabolic rate than a sedentary person, thereby resulting in more utilization of energy. The active person may have a higher resting metabolism as well, which means that he or she may be able to consume just as many calories as an inactive person and not gain weight when the other does. This is sometimes referred to as a fast or high metabolism. The resting metabolic rate is also related to the surface area of the body. As weight increases, the amount of energy needed to keep basic bodily functions running increases. This means that an overweight person's body perceives that he or she needs more energy and thereby conserves it. The way to change the metabolic rate is to become more active.

Unfortunately, many obese people do not expend much energy. In fact you may notice a slow-motion quality about them that looks even restful without much twitching and fidgeting. Even these tiny movements, however, burn energy. Exercise, a word that conjures up intense fears and revulsion in many, is one of the most crucial ingredients in weight loss. Frequently, the overweight individual detests exercise, but *any* movement is precisely what is necessary in long-term success of weight loss.

Metabolic requirements also vary with age. The highest rate of energy intake per body weight in humans is required by infants. There is a gradual decline in childhood and further decline in adult life. Metabolic rates for women are usually lower than those for men, so women may need to consume less calories except during pregnancy and lactation, when energy demands increase. Although there are calorie charts available for review, there is considerable variation in these energy requirements, even for individuals of the same size, age, and sex. For example, for a 130 pound, moderately active woman, the caloric requirement is approximately 2,000 calories. However, there may be as much as a 20 percent variation for women with the same activity level and body size.

Recent findings in the medical literature on mechanisms in the development and maintenance of obesity have focused not on just the consequence of eating too much, but also on expending too little energy. Two recent medical studies on the development of obesity in infancy and adulthood suggest that differences in activity may be the key point in obesity. In one study, clinical investigators measured the total seven-day energy intake and energy expenditure of a group of infants, aged three months, and related their results to weight gain during the first year of life. The data indicates that infants who are overweight on their first birthday have a 20.7 percent lower expenditure of energy than infants who are of normal weight. The two groups do not differ significantly in energy intake. These findings suggest that both activity level and food intake are critical in determining weight gain at an early age but the former appears to be more significant. *An increase in physical activity will expend more energy and is probably more important in weight reduction than caloric intake.* So the first awareness in losing weight is to think in terms of achieving a negative energy balance.

SOLVING THE WEIGHT–GAIN MYSTERY

It was once believed that the major cause for obesity was overeating. But if this were true, the easiest way to lose weight would be to eat less. As this is not so easy, it is clearly not the whole story. The causes of weight gain are numerous, multifactorial, and complex. These include genetic, environmental, and psychosocial factors, as well as individual differences in eating patterns, resting metabolic rate, biochemical shifts, and the unusual phenomenon of "brown fat."

Brown fat is more metabolically active than stored fat and actually has the ability to burn energy, turning excess calories into heat production. This is believed, for example, to be a major factor in the dissipation of heat in hibernating animals. Some researchers believe that thin people who eat excessively and yet are not overly active may have a larger quantity of brown fat in proportion to stored fat, resulting in a greater expenditure of energy. We all know individuals who seemingly "eat all they want" and yet remain thin despite the fact that they are not overly active. Brown fat may be the secret to this mystery. (Many people, however, do not have much brown fat and, quite the opposite, have an undesirable storage of adipose tissue or body fat.)

Overwhelming research indicates that all of these factors, in combination with a lifestyle of inactivity, appear to be the core factors in weight gain. Consider the fact, as we have mentioned previously, that it takes approximately 100 calories of energy to walk one mile. If we walk one mile a day, we will have an energy output of 700 calories per week.

Multiply this times 52 weeks and our calorie expenditure per year will equal 36,400 calories. Since a pound of fat contains approximately 3,500 calories, this daily one mile walk is equivalent to the loss of approximately ten pounds of fat in one year, if all other factors remain equal. Thus, by simple mathematics, it becomes clear how this whole energetic concept works in obesity and weight gain.

Caloric intake (what you eat) is another major consideration in weight loss. When the caloric intake is below the daily energy requirement, the initial loss in body weight results primarily from a depletion in the body's carbohydrate stores. In continued weight loss, body fat is metabolized and, therefore, required to supply the caloric deficiency. In other words, by *restricting food intake and/or by increasing physical activity, the body burns up fat.* Fad diets, however, are the opposite. These are diets that tend to fool the body's biochemistry by manipulating proteins, carbohydrates, or fat. These types of diets are nutritionally unbalanced, usually advocating levels of high protein, with and without high fat intake, and low carbohydrate consumption. In the late 1970's, such diets were found to be associated with cardiac arrhythmias and even sudden death.

The once popular ketogenic diet, such as the Atkins diet, employed a high protein, high-fat/low-carbohydrate regimen to achieve rapid weight loss. Since these diets are largely composed of eating fat with very little glucose, the body relies on the breakdown of fat for its metabolic function. This results in a high blood level of free fatty acids which are insufficiently burned, thus producing ketones. Ketones make the blood more acid, resulting in loss of appetite. The Scarsdale Diet also was based on eating a diet high in protein and low in fat. In this case the body metabolizes its own fat, not only from adipose (fat) tissue, but other tissues as well. If you consume excessive protein, however, especially while not exercising, this can be converted to fat, and may actually work against your weight-loss goals. Although these diets may cause initial weight loss, it is done at the expense of the body. Besides these diets are unnatural and one cannot tolerate them for long. The most effective nutritional programs are those that are balanced with proper amounts of carbohydrates and proteins.

A low-fat/high-fiber concept is the most scientifically sound concept. Some dietary programs include fasting, seemingly the diet of choice during the 1980s. While this may be a good way to start weight loss, I believe such an involvement requires close medical supervision with continual follow-up investigation while evaluating sound nutritional principles. In addition, a long-term involvement with behavioral modification is still necessary to prevent the old patterns from re-emerging. This was the case in our hospital-based program. Although most participants lost more than 40 pounds of weight, many of them regained the weight. Weight reduction needs long-term commitment, emotional support, and psychological awareness.

CHAPTER 3

AT THE HEART OF THE MATTER

This book is designed to give you valuable tools to effectively and permanently transform your relationship with your body. Of course, a beneficial result is that you will have a trimmer, more physically fit, healthier body. But the deeper more profound transformation is about your relationship with yourself. This requires a physical, mental, and emotional shift. If you now find yourself criticizing your body, condemning yourself, feeling self-hate, or hurting yourself, working through these core emotional issues and getting to the heart of the matter will free you.

Weight loss comes out of healing the relationship between the body and the mind. The results of healing your inner conflicts will be a self-acceptance, self-love, and a sense of truly honoring your body. Using a holistic approach to weight loss prevents using dieting as yet another unhealthy neurotic expression of an unresolved self. The vicious cycle of hating your body, going on a diet, losing weight, gaining the weight back, hating yourself and your body must be interrupted and healed. These are habits disrespectful to yourself.

A holistic approach does not mean you have to go on a vegetarian diet or become spiritual. It simply means that the approach to permanent body changes is multilevel: emotional, behavioral, physical, and nutritional. In the overweight syndrome, we create negative feelings about ourselves and our bodies. Emotional factors such as depression, helplessness, guilt, loneliness, boredom, self-hate, denial of anger, fear, and hopelessness are meshed in this cycle.

IT'S TIME TO REFRAME

But let's reframe your attitude toward your body and weight loss. The concept of "reframing" is to redefine negative attitudes and beliefs, some of which we learned as young children, in a more positive light. Reframing results in seeing the good aspect of any given situation or person including ourselves. For example, let's reframe your attitude toward your body and weight loss. Let's see your overweight condition as a gift because it is now the impetus for you to delve deeper into your psyche and into the blocks that have hampered your self-image and self-esteem. You can use it as a motivating force to heal deep emotional issues, become more alive, and live a more pleasurable, fulfilling life free of obsessive-complusive behavior.

What a joy life can be when your thought process is free from a preoccupation with your body and/or your food. After all, what we think, we can internalize and begin to believe. What we believe, we become. If we think we have an unattractive body, for example, and think it often, we believe we are unattractive and thus may act in an unattractive manner. This negativity limits the vast possibilities of experience. Whereas if we reframe this view, we will consciously look at ourselves in a constructive, not destructive, way. In other words, we can now look at our beautiful hair or bright eyes and see ourselves attractively. This does not mean we should stay stuck in fat bodies, but we should use positive reframing as a tool to get past this unconscious block.

For people who are chronically overweight, food becomes a vehicle with which to block the emotions. In the book, *Overcoming Overeating*, by Jane R. Hirschmann and Carol H. Munter, the authors make a distinction between stomach hunger and mouth hunger. When you eat in order to fill your body because your stomach is hungry, you are in a healthy relationship with food. If you find yourself wanting food out of mouth hunger, even when you are not hungry, you are experiencing something emotional, an anxiety out of conscious awareness; that is, you are using food to try to assuage, hide, or substitute for the feeling. I agree with this theory. For example, perhaps we are feeling deep despair or intense rage, but these feelings do not feel safe. We then feel anxiety about having these feelings. If we are not getting in touch with our true feelings and expressing them, overeating may be a futile attempt to sublimate whatever the true feeling is.

Another example might be love. A lot of us can give but cannot receive. We may not be able to take in love, but we can take in food. Therefore, we use food as a substitute for emotional and spiritual hunger. Afterwards, we get upset and scold ourselves for binging and being fat, though it is not the food that is the problem but what it represents. It is what food substitutes for that people *really* need to examine. Food may be used as a drug. Like alcohol, we medicate ourselves with it, especially sugar, but it never cures the problem. It exacerbates it. It continues. And the reality is that we physically feed ourselves to death while we *emotionally starve* ourselves to death. What a paradox!

The cause of eating disorders, addictive behavior, and obsessive-compulsive patterns often stem from a variety of painful experiences in childhood, frequently combined with bad habits that were taught in the family system. Unless we are actively involved (through support groups and workshops, therapy or a personal search) in uncovering the causes, the core issues remain, although unconscious. A powerful beginning is to get in touch with our own experience; that is, to bring out of darkness and into the light our own unconscious motivations for overeating.

WORMS ARE GOOD!

You may be thinking, "I don't need to do that. My body may be a problem, but not my mind. Why open a can of worms?" However, as a physician, I know that the body speaks the truth and the mind can be deceived. I choose to trust the body. The body reacts to repressed emotion. Unfortunately, most parents do not teach children to honor or express their emotions, and they give many mixed messages about very natural human aspects of their physical being. Children are told, "Stop crying," when they are hurt and have a need to cry. They are told that anger is not ladylike or that men should not be afraid. Many people have been treated disrespectfully and abusively (physically or emotionally) through the years and have come to view this treatment as normal, acceptable, and to be expected and even deserved. As children, some would even get hit, emotionally abused, reprimanded, or abandoned when they expressed certain emotions such as anger, sadness, or fear. Alice Miller, author of *The Drama of the Gifted Child,* tells us that parents unknowingly have the power to form and deform the emotional and physical lives of their children.

We were all born with the natural ability to release emotion. If we watch a baby who is upset, we will see that he or she will cry or scream and that when finished, the body softens and the baby is peaceful and smiling again. However, if the baby is misdirected from its natural pattern, this may result in lifelong repression of feelings. Where does all this repressed emotional energy go? It becomes an unresolved memory in the unconscious. The energy actually gets stuck in the body, in the muscles and in the cells. This unreleased energy becomes the seat of "dis-ease" and "dis-harmony" inside of us.

DOWN MEMORY LANE

For you to begin to lose weight, it is very important to take an honest look at how your parents related to you in terms of food, diet, your emotional needs, and your self-image. This may be a painful look. Be aware that you might have some denial systems blocking you from seeing the truth, but it is worth a try. This is why support groups can be so helpful when attempting to lose weight. What feelings were you not allowed to have as a child? Were you told to stop crying when you were sad? Did you get punished? Were you taught to control yourself, control your feelings? Were your parents controlling about what you ate and how much you ate? Did they force you to eat everything that was on your plate, even if you were full? Take some time to look back at their belief systems about food and about body size. Did your parents believe that "a fat baby is a healthy baby?" Were you ever given the message that if you didn't eat, you would get sick? Were there reward systems set up around food? If you were hungry and wanted to eat, did you ever hear the familiar phrase, as written by Hirschmann and Zaphiropoulos in *Are You Hungry,* "don't spoil your appetite," a refrain heard by each generation of growing children?

What does it mean? How can anyone "spoil" an appetite by eating? Appetite is an internal signal; hunger pangs indicate a need for food. Eating satisfies, not spoils an appetite. What parents really mean when they say this is that the child should stifle his or her appetite, or natural feelings of hunger, in order to please the parent. They mean, "Don't eat when and what you want to eat, but eat when and what I want you to eat."

A powerful way to heal the wounds that we all carry from childhood is to be able to now express what we wanted to express back then, but couldn't. This is best done in therapy or in some other safe environment. In this way, we will be able to diffuse the old feelings that we have about past events and not apply them to current situations. In other words, once an old feeling is released, when a new experience causes us to react emotionally, it won't contain the charge or the excess baggage of all the other past repressed feelings. Therefore, the present feeling will be more manageable, the anxiety lessened, and your need to turn to food will be considerably assuaged.

It is important to allow negative emotions to come up so they can be released and yet it is also important to reframe them. This may sound like a contradiction. How do you know when to do what? The rule is to first EXPERIENCE the feeling without judgment or self-editorialization, and then to investigate it once it has been discharged. For example, let's say you constantly insult your body. You can feel how angry you really are at yourself. You have been feeling these particular feelings for quite some time and the intense emotional charge must be expressed and released. Take some time privately or perhaps in a therapy session to vent this anger.

Once you do this (perhaps you'll need to do this every so often for a while), you can eventually try to understand the roots of this behavior. It will then be easier to catch yourself saying or thinking something self-destructive so you can reframe it in a positive light. This process can be particularly effective in losing weight. When you find yourself reaching for food when you are not hungry, rather than eating right away, sit down with a pen and a pad and write what you are feeling or immediately express these feelings verbally. In this way you derail the maladaptive motivation behind the mouth hunger.

TAKE SUCCESSFUL SMALL STEPS

It is important to point out here the need for patience. If you want to successfully change your patterns it will take time, repetition, and a tremendous amount of patience. Realize that you are taking a totally new approach to reshaping your body. Let go of any sense of time and urgency. Relax. Pushing too hard and forcing the flow will create a destructive, frenetic energy about this process. People want fast results, fast cures, and immediate gratification, but I am a firm believer in taking out the struggle and in not driving ourselves beyond normal capacity. Healing unhealthy and destructive patterns requires focus, time and energy. So patience, lots of nurturing and self-love and self-support are necessary here. It is healthful to let go of preconceived notions of how much weight you have to lose and in what span of time. Expectations, after all, can lead to disappointments. This can then trigger a sense of failure and a vicious cycle of obsessive eating.

A major pitfall in losing weight is creating an unattainable goal. Our society has placed a tremendous pressure on us to be beautiful. The model we have been given for beauty is a thin body. But we must all get to a place where we feel a sense of peace about our particular body types. There is indeed a danger in seeking total perfection, as it is truly an unattainable goal. Perhaps you are bottom heavy and overweight, but you begin to make changes in your lifestyle and you start to reduce. You are exercising and firming up and looking much slimmer, much better. If you continue to focus on your heavy thighs, however, you create a counterproductive attitude. Instead of feeling and expressing a tremendous gratitude toward yourself for reshaping your body, an expression which will encourage your entire being to continue to change your patterns, you are busy putting yourself down for "heavy thighs." This creates a futile, rebellious feeling inside. A part of you will be feeling "Why bother? No matter what I do, it's never enough."

SEX?

In this multi-level approach to creating and maintaining a new body, it is very important to establish a beneficial goal. If you want to change your body in order to have a healthy body/mind connection, your focus is in the right place. If your reasons for losing weight are that you think if you do so you will get love, or so-and-so will want you or envy you, or you'll get that job or someone to pay attention to you, etc., you are setting yourself up to fail. This can be an unfulfilled expectation. What if you lose the weight and it doesn't happen? Or, what if you lose the weight and it does happen, but you still feel unfulfilled? The way to protect yourself from an unfulfilled prophecy is to set your sights on a beneficial intention. "When my lifestyle patterns change, when I have a healthier relationship to myself and my body, I will feel more alive, more at peace and, therefore, I will experience more pleasure." If you can begin to see yourself in a healing process and feel a sense of hope and excitement about it, you can begin to enjoy the process rather than being caught up in the end result. Let go of the struggle, or the "I'll be happy when…" syndrome.

Liken this venture to reprogramming a computer. There are many circuits. Some circuits are emotional blocks, some are faulty belief systems, some are negative family patterns, some are your own destructive habits, and on and on. Where have you been short-circuited? What experiences have caused you to cut off from yourself? All this must be worked on in order to heal yourself and your unconscious obsession with food. The unconscious drives are stronger than the conscious drives. It is frequently the unconscious desires that direct us. Thus, to begin to enjoy food and feel we have permission to eat, we must be at peace with ourselves emotionally. There is often a direct correlation between anxiety and overeating. If understanding ourselves better and feeling that we are actively involved in our own healing reduces anxiety, it will have a positive effect on healing the eating compulsion. When we bring aspects of our unconsciousness into the light of awareness, they are no longer hidden forces and we begin to have a greater ability to not let them control and harm us. If overeating is a negative way to cope with feelings, especially feelings of fear or powerlessness, then creating a better relationship with the emotional self will significantly support the healing of this compulsion.

This was probably the case with Roger Buffaloe who must have had feelings of powerlessness, most likely rooted in his childhood. By becoming a successful businessman, he established the *Image* of success which gave him a sense of control. He obviously did not have this in his eating habits. The truth is, he was out of control. This is a typical scenario of many obese individuals, male and female. With women, there may be even a greater risk of obesity because of their lack of early support to express themselves emotionally and physically, and particularly because of their feelings of vulnerability.

What I want to help you get in touch with now is the fearful side of weight loss. Both men and women have concern about this deep core issue, sexual vulnerability. To get in touch with your own feelings about this, write or say out loud the following and take your time to fill in the blanks:

"If I lose weight I'm afraid… will happen."

"If I lose weight I'm afraid… (who) will pull away from me."

"If I lose weight, I'm afraid I'll hurt… "

"By being overweight I feel protected from… "

"By being overweight I don't have to deal with… "

"If I have a sexier body I'm afraid… "

While I was a therapist in the hospital-wide weight loss program at Manchester Memorial Hospital in Connecticut, it became increasingly clear to me that the issue of sexuality was a major factor in the over-weight syndrome. Many of my OptiFast weight-loss clients communicated their intense fears regarding weight loss. There were also issues of love and relationship. For example, one of my clients said, "By eating, I will make myself so unlovable that I will never get hurt again." She had deep, painful issues regarding love and sexuality. For some of my clients, losing weight was like shedding "suits of armor." The physical padding that being overweight provides can be viewed as a protective armor. This maladaptive defense mechanism, unconsciously created to avoid pain, actually holds past pain deep inside your tissues. Are you unconsciously or consciously holding on to the weight to protect your-self sexually? Do you use the weight to avoid other forms of intimacy? It is important to honestly delve into these possibilities because unless they are uncovered and dealt with emotionally, it will be very difficult to reduce and keep the weight off. To shed the armor makes us vulner-able. It is this shedding of armor and the ensuing vulnerability that is for some a major cause of resistance in losing further weight. Let me give you an example.

SEXUAL VIOLATION MAY CAUSE WEIGHT GAIN

One of the ladies in my program lost 30–40 pounds. She was quite intuitive about herself, particularly since she had been in psychothera-py. After the miraculous weight loss, however, she became blocked and actually started to gain weight. She told us she was "sick of the diet." She was putting up tremendous resistance. I asked her if anything was wrong and she said she had no problems. But there was a problem. The body told the truth in that she started to put on weight. So I asked again what was going on with her. She told me she wanted to go back to her old manner of eating. Then I asked her what was going on with her relationship with her husband. At that point she froze. She looked at me and she started to cry and then said, "I'm very scared." She communicated to me that her husband was looking at her with a new energy. It was an energy that she did not feel comfortable with and yet did not know why. As he approached her with this new energy, she became more and more frightened and was afraid of his sexual advances. She remembered these looks from when she was a little girl. Although she had been in therapy before, she never worked on sexual issues. For some reason both she and her therapist did not feel that this was important. Unfortunately, sexual issues are frequently avoided by the client as well as the therapist. In fact, this woman had been wounded as a child. She, indeed, had a history of subtle sexual violation. Although this did not appear to be overt; that is, she did not appear to have recollection of any childhood abuse or molestation, she did feel an uneasiness about a masculine drive and sexual advance.

Previously, I quoted Alice Miller's work in discussing how parents unknowingly, and the key word here is unknowingly, cross a boundary that has a sexual connotation. A five-year-old child cannot distinguish between love and sexuality. Love and sexuality are the same thing for a five-year-old child. When a child sits on her father's lap, for example, and enjoys the warmth and love of cuddling and then wants to leave, this is a way of satisfying her need for simple contact and then her need for separation. This is a common phenomenon in children.

However, if the father frequently uses his daughter as an object for his own need for contact, this is crossing a boundary. The child feels this intrusion energetically, which is also transferred into the unconscious and later experienced as a sexual taboo or a fear of subsequent sexual contact. But where does one leave off and the other begin? Aren't fathers naturally loving toward their children, some more enthusiastically than others? I believe incest issues nowadays can be seen as fashionable and overplayed, but crossing boundaries can be very subtle and, in most cases, unconscious. Loving and genuine affectionate feelings for a child are the reality of human nature. The trap for both the parents and the child is that the unfulfilled need for contact in the adult is acted out on the child rather than the parents finding it in their own relationships.

Of course, there are also more overt cases of sexual abuse which include not only seduction but molestation, incest, and rape. While not all overweight people have been sexually abused as children, abundant medical literature indicates that eating disorders are a frequent result of sexual abuse. Symptoms found in incest and rape victims include fear, sleeping and eating disturbances, as well as sexual dysfunction. Obesity and compulsive eating are ways that survivors of childhood abuse protect themselves. Overeating and putting on weight as body armor can be a way to avoid unwanted sexual advances and thus become less vulnerable.

Although many clients in psychotherapy do not remember overt or covert sexual abuse, the body does remember. For example, a powerful female colleague of mine told me that several years ago she had a severe weight problem. While today she is an attractive woman at 5 feet, 7 inches, weighing approximately 125 pounds, she used to weight 180 pounds. She communicated to me that in her college days and particularly in graduate school when she was training to become a massage therapist, she was very heavy and heavily armored. She did not know why. She had an obsession with food that she did not understand. She also related to me that she had the feeling that she was molested as a child though she didn't know how, nor could she remember the circumstances. When she was working on her own body as a massage therapist, the memories began to come back. She saw a counselor and she reconstructed some of the forgotten memories of childhood. Although she could not put it completely together, she said that there was a feeling of aggressive male energy that was sexual in nature when she was a young girl. When she went to college, she got involved in a very passionate relationship, and this brought up the previous unpleasant experience of male energy coming toward her as a defenseless young child.

At that point she started to put on weight. She gained approximately 50 pounds, becoming less attractive. After she gained her insight and the awareness that her sexuality was the key to her obesity, she began to cry and cry and cry. She grieved for months. She knew how important crying was and used it as a healing modality. After this long process of grieving, she became in touch with her true self and began to lose the weight in an easy and timely manner. She now is able to help others who have been in similar situations.

Unrecognized fear, in addition to sadness and anger, creates forces in our personality that unconsciously make us eat. It is not uncommon to find that the root of an individual's weight problem is prior sexual abuse, which may be obvious in some and not so obvious in others. It is also a simple fact that some people just like to eat. Not everyone has a hidden sexual issue as an origin to their weight problem. As a matter of fact, the converse was true in another of my clients. Jean had a strong sexual desire that she found imprisoned in her body.

After losing approximately 40 pounds, however, she developed a feeling of freedom about her sexuality. This realization occurred in one of her dreams. She dreamed that her whole body was encased in an orthopedic cast. It suddenly started to crack from the front to the back. As her body armor was falling apart, she found herself in the bathroom with a naked man – a symbol of sexuality. She communicated that she had good feelings in the dream. She in fact liked the dream. She did not experience fear. What she was experiencing was a new emergence of feelings of aliveness and vitality. She was excited about her new body and the way she looked. Her self-image was improving and she was looking forward to experiencing her new awareness of sexuality. Jean's dream was, indeed, a signal of emotional healing.

The need for emotional healing is a global one. In our particular society, we have not been given tools with which to understand our emotions. On the contrary, our society has negated the value of emotions and judged certain emotions as weak or inappropriate. It considers strength to be holding yourself up and being strong. This is not true strength if we are "just acting" strong while inside we don't feel strong at all. People have become afraid of emotions and tend to feel uncomfortable when around someone who is crying deeply. It is felt as dangerous and threatening. We have all been taught to cut off from and repress our feelings and have not been given healthy ways to release pent up emotional energy. The following are a *few tools that will help bring about the emotional healing that will aid in developing greater self-esteem and subsequent weight loss.*

Breathing

When we are afraid, anxious, or nervous, we hold our breath. Due to the high level of stress in living, unfortunately, most people don't breathe deeply enough. Faced with a fight or flight trauma, a simple deep breath can sometimes save lives. It brings our focus of attention back to the immediate and grounds us in our bodies. The best way to become aware of our own need to breathe is to watch for signs of anxiety. Wanting to eat, even though we are not hungry, may be an overt sign of an unconscious motivation that deep breathing could assuage. Some of us may reach for a cigarette or an alcoholic drink. Again, deep breathing can sometimes get us through the crucial point when we are about to do something self-destructive. A more prolonged form of breathing is meditation. If you are not ready to meditate, or don't feel it is for you, however, you will benefit by simply taking time out of each day to sit quietly and breathe deeply and slowly. Making contact with your body through breath is an important part of reconnecting with yourself.

MEDITATION

Meditation is easy to learn. The most difficult part may be finding the time. But creating the time, whether it be every day or three times a week, can be rewarding, offering you growth and insight. You might feel tremendous resistance or fear of doing it wrong, but there is no one set way to meditate. Often, the biggest obstacle is our own judgment that we are not really in a meditative state. The mere fact that we have taken 5 minutes or 45 minutes to sit or lie quietly and breathe, however, is meditative in itself. Don't compare yourself to others' accounts of their meditations. If your quiet time doesn't measure up to how you perceive meditation to be, you run the risk of thinking you failed. As you practice it more and more, you will find that your body quiets down more easily.

In order to do this, you must go to a room where you won't be interrupted. Put the answering machine on. Sit in a comfortable chair or lie down on a carpet with a small pillow (optional) under your head. If this is the first time you are attempting meditation, your body might find five reasons why you have to pop up and do something. You might lie down and feel very fidgety. Close your eyes. Start by taking five slow breaths in and out through the mouth. Tell yourself to relax. Continue to breathe slowly and deeply, either in through the nose and out the mouth, or in and out through the nose, whichever is more comfortable. Feel your body. Put your consciousness in your head and slowly, as you breathe, run your consciousness down your body. If you are having trouble relaxing, tell each part of your body to relax by saying, "My head is relaxed, my legs are relaxed, etc,". Many thoughts might run through your head. Don't resist them, but don't focus on them. Merely note them and let them pass. You may imagine opening a door and saying to all these thoughts, "I know you're there, but I don't want to let you in." See or feel these thoughts going out the door and close the door behind them. You may need to do this a few times.

When you feel you are relaxed enough, you will begin breathing naturally. Take in slow deep breaths every so often, and remember to let the air out slowly. Imagine that you have an inner physician. This inner healer is very wise and loving and may be called upon for a vast supply of ideas and information. Tell it all about your pain, particularly about your body. Let yourself flow with this process. See what you need to express to this inner healer and then ask it for help or guidance. State, for example, that you want to attract the perfect support system. Know that you have a right to ask for this. If you feel sadness, let yourself cry. Whatever you feel, allow it completely. Stay open to receive insights, but don't struggle. Just trust that guidance will come in various ways. For example, you might be in the shower later and feel inspired to call someone to establish a connection. Einstein supposedly got his best ideas while in the shower and relaxing. Follow whatever instincts you may have. When you feel complete, take a few more breaths. Slowly open your eyes.

You can also use meditation to reframe your self-image. If you have been overweight for many years, you may be holding onto a self-defeating image as a "fat person" who is doomed to a lifetime of being fat and/or struggling with fat. Go into a deep relaxation and remember to breathe deeply and take your time. When you are deep in relaxation, start to ask yourself to bring forth all your fears about your own body image. For example, you may fear that you will never have the pleasure of a thinner body. But affirm to yourself that you will by saying, "I will become thin." Take deep breaths as you do this. When you feel complete, start to work on the self-image you would like to have. Tell yourself that you can indeed change your body. You can change destructive patterns. Remind yourself that other people have done it, and you can too! Take some time to visualize yourself feeling healthier, lighter, stronger, and filled with vitality. Remember, repetition is very important in shifting your belief systems and your attitude. Working your mind on a deep level will aid the momentum of this reprogramming process.

EMOTIONAL EXERCISES

Another essential door to unlock is getting in touch with the various conflicts you may be holding onto unconsciously in terms of having a trimmer body. You can either do this sitting down with a paper and pen or by releasing them verbally or physically, as I will describe. There are many different exercises you can do. For example, when you feel very sad, try to lie down, tilt your head back, and let down into the feelings. Get deep into sobbing. The more your cry from your abdomen, the better the releasing. As you are in this state, try to get in touch with the grieving you have had during your struggle. Crying is the most healing of all the emotions. If you feel angry, however, or enraged, try yelling or screaming while in your car. Remember to roll up the windows so you feel private and safe. Or, go out to the woods or a secluded beach and scream at the person whom you are feeling angry toward. Get it all out. Say everything you feel without editing your language. Because he or she is not present, this is your opportunity to release the energy. You could also take a tennis racket and physically hit your bed and scream.

Another good exercise is to lie on your bed and just kick. By kicking and screaming and shaking your head, you can simulate a temper tantrum. Other forms of anger-release work include making a fist and jutting out your jaw in defiance or protest. Another way is to twist a towel and release a sound while your are doing it. There are forms of therapy that teach you how to release your emotions using safe, private, effective, and beneficial techniques.

Many people may find it difficult, however, to start to release the years of pent-up emotional energy alone. It is a sign of great strength to realize you want to help yourself. This may include doing emotional release work alone at home, or in a safe place such as a therapist's office. It is important to release the core of your sadness, your anger, and your fears one way or another. When this happens, we begin to get in touch with our true needs and really experience our true selves. This is a significant step in the right direction and a profound step in the *Lose to Win* philosophy.

CHAPTER 4

THE NUTS AND BOLTS OF NUTRITION

In order to eat nutritionally, it's important that you understand some basics about how food affects your body. Although some of this information may be more than you care to know right now, I hope you'll find yourself referring back to this chapter again and again.

Remember that the loss of excess fat results from a negative energy balance and energy is derived from calories. Food calories can be divided into three major components: proteins, carbohydrates, and fats, with alcohol being a fourth less important contributor. When counting calories we need to consider the percentages that come from proteins, carbohydrates, or fats in any given serving.

Each of these nutrients provides different amounts of energy (calories per gram or per ounce) measured through sophisticated clinical studies. The following provides useful values for comparison: Carbohydrates contain four calories per gram or 112 calories per ounce; fats contain nine calories per gram or 232 calories per ounce; proteins contain four calories per gram or 112 calories per ounce. From this brief analysis, one can easily see that an individual can eat over twice as many carbohydrates or proteins as fats and still have the same caloric intake. Alcohol has seven calories per gram or 196 calories per ounce, which is usually only one cocktail.

Foods are classified according to their calorie density. For example, three ounces of fish contains approximately 150 calories, which is less than three ounces of beef chuck, which contains approximately 300 calories. Such caloric densities are usually related to the amount of fat in the food. Fish contains relatively less fat than beef. Therefore, more fish can be eaten than beef for the same amount of calories. But more fish may not be needed to satisfy hunger, so one can reduce total intake and, therefore, lose weight.

We can see that it is important to know the fat content in food. Being nutritionally aware is to choose foods that provide the most nutrition with the fewest fats and calories. For example, whole milk is approximately 50 percent fat while one percent milk is approximately 18 percent fat. If most of us can make the gradual transition from whole milk to one percent milk, the amount of calories is reduced by nearly half. One percent milk is less calorie-dens, and, therefore, more healthy. And remember the cardinal rule: *No deprivation and no loss of pleasure.*

Such a weight-loss program may not only be one that is calorie-dilute but also one that contains healthy amounts of carbohydrates, proteins, and fats. In considering a healthy diet or a healthy lifestyle we again have to remember that deprivation is the oppositional force. When putting our meals together we strive for a reasonable balance of carbohydrates, proteins, and fats, but do we know how to do this properly? The rule of thumb is surprisingly simple: *Approximately 65 to 70 percent of the diet should be complex carbohydrates while 10 to 15 percent of the daily intake should include proteins, with the remaining calories coming from fat.* But why eat fat at all?

The body requires essential fatty acids for normal functioning and most foods, including some vegetables, have at least 15 percent of their total calories in fat. The American Heart Association recommends 30 percent of the dietary intake from fats, but I think 15 to 20 percent is adequate. The real problem in lowering fat content in the diet is that fat simply tastes good. Although now many Americans are fat conscious, most of our diets still approach a fat content making up approximately 40 to 50 percent of our daily intake. Considering that the American Heart Association recommends that fat intake be less than 30 percent of the total calories and the famous Pritikin diet, which some cardiologists endorse, only has five to ten percent of the total calories coming from fat, I think we can find a reasonable balance that is neither too strict nor depriving of pleasure.

NUTRITIONAL AWARENESS KEEPS POUNDS OFF, FAT OUT

Medical research indicates that weight gain is not only related to the total number of calories but also to the total number of grams of fat in the diet. Reducing our intake of fat is a cardinal ingredient in weight loss and good health. Generally, people have considerable resistance to reducing the fat intake in their diets. However, it is crucial to point out that fat intake should be kept to a minimum to maximize weight loss and ensure a health conscious lifestyle. In considering a nutritional awareness program, and particularly in losing weight, it is important to focus our attention on the number of grams of fat in our daily consumption. This can be done by reading labels and avoiding various cooking techniques that result in excess fat content.

Mushrooms, for example, contain approximately less than ten percent of their calories in fat, but if they are deep fried in oil or if they are broiled in butter, the calorie content is considerably higher. Onions are approximately three to five percent fat, but fried as onion rings, the fat content approaches 90 percent. Again, this is calorie-dense and a poor choice when seeking a healthy, nutritional balance.

In calculating the percentage of fat in a particular product, you must know the calories per serving and the number of grams of fat per serving. The calculation process goes something like this: Multiply the number of grams of fat by nine (remember there are nine calories per gram of fat) to determine the total number of fat calories in a food product. Next, divide the number of fat calories by the number of total calories in the serving. Now convert this to a percentage by multiplying by 100. (grams fat x 9 divided by cal/serving x 100 =) The goal in losing weight and staying healthy is to primarily choose foods that are approximately less than 20 percent fat.

Let's now focus attention on the calculations of carbohydrates and proteins. One has to keep in mind that each gram of protein or carbohydrate has four calories. The calculation for caloric value in proteins and carbohydrates is similar to fat content, but then we need to multiply by four instead of nine. Then divide the number of protein or carbohydrate calories by the number of calories per serving and again convert this to a percentage (multiply by 100). With simple arithmetic, one can determine the percent of calories of protein, carbohydrate, and fat in a particular food. For example, potato chips are approximately 60 percent fat. For the usual serving of ten potato chips there is approximately 115 calories, one gram of protein, ten grams of carbohydrates, and eight grams of fat per serving.

To determine the percentage of fat, remember our formula requiring two crucial pieces of information: (1) The total number of calories per serving; (2) The grams of fat per serving. Therefore, multiply eight grams of fat by nine calories per gram and this equals 72 calories. Next, divide the number of fat calories by the number of total calories, which is 72 over 115. Now convert this to a percentage by multiplying by 100. The figure comes out to 62.6 percent of its calories from fat. Since potato chips contain such a considerable quantity of fat, in this case even a small portion is detrimental to diet and health. At 115 calories and 8 grams of fat for ten chips, just imagine *how many calories you can consume sitting with a bowl of chips watching television and not even feel satisfied.* It is important to understand that substituting foods that give us the same satisfaction but less fat content and consequently less weight gain will alleviate the feelings of hunger. Again, our most important tool in losing weight is knowledge and awareness of the fat content in our diets.

Protein and carbohydrate awareness is equally important. The American population is highly preoccupied with the seeming need for protein. Meat and potatoes for most of us was our typical diet growing up. We all have heard the stories of how meat is necessary for protein in our diet and for strong and healthy bodies. Yes, it is true that meat provides a major source of protein, but how much protein do we really need?

Ordinarily, most scientists are in agreement that approximately one gram of protein is necessary per kilogram (2.2 pounds) of body weight per day. Therefore, a 150 pound sedentary man needs approximately 55 to 65 grams of protein per day. If we consume enough calories, however, excess proteins will be converted to fat and stored in the body to be burned later for energy. Since a man of this size consumes approximately 2,400 calories per day, then recommended protein consumption should approximate 12 percent of his dietary calories. But if this individual were to eat more protein, as opposed to carbohydrates, much of the excess protein would be stored as fat. Since most Americans consume approximately one and a half to two times as much protein as they need, this is an easy and often overlooked source of weight gain.

YOU AND YOUR BUN

The process of converting protein (amino acids) into fat is called deamination. This can cause considerable metabolic stress to the body. During this process the nitrogen that is released from the amino acids is quickly converted into ammonia. Since ammonia is toxic to the body, this is changed into the breakdown product called urea. Blood urea nitrogen, or BUN, is a measure of the kidney function and really is a product of the breakdown of nitrogen waste products in the body. In a normal balanced diet where protein consists of approximately 10 to 15 percent of the total caloric intake, our bodies can easily dispose of the urea through the normal functioning of the kidneys. However, if we take in excess quantities of protein, such as 20 to 25 percent, this will cause a buildup of urea, which needs water for metabolism. If we do not drink enough water, our bodies take it from our tissues to dilute the urea, placing an enormous burden on the kidneys.

Such a scenario occurs in individuals on very high protein diets. Wrestlers trying to "make weight" frequently use this destructive technique. This was the case with myself during my college career, when as a wrestler I needed to maintain a weight approximately 10 to 12 pounds lighter than my natural and healthy weight. Our coaches recommended a high protein diet – and we wondered why we were continuously "dying of thirst!" Yes, I was able to make the weight on every occasion, but this was at the expense of my renal or kidney function. After nine years of wrestling through high school and college, my kidney function was slightly abnormal when I entered medical school. The excess toxicities induced by high protein metabolism, coupled with a poor intake of fluid, probably affected the status of my kidneys. It is important for you to understand that healthy weight loss needs to be accomplished without a manipulation of proteins and carbohydrates. Unknowingly, I caused renal dysfunction in myself, which could have been extremely hazardous. Lucky for me I stopped the "protein diet" before it had the time to do lasting damage. Protein, though, has many important functions in the body. It makes up the muscles, ligaments, tendons, organs, glands, nails, hair, and some body fluids. Proteins are also essential for growth. Amino acids are essential in building healthy muscles.

Amino acids are the building blocks of protein. Because protein is composed of different acids, each amino acid has a specific function. There are two types of amino acids – the essential and the nonessential. The nonessential amino acids can be produced by the liver and include approximately 80 percent of the amino acids we need. The remaining 20 percent must be obtained from outside sources. There are nine essential amino acids. If we do not consume foods with enough of the essential amino acids, the body may be unable to produce the protein it requires for healthy functioning. We all have seen signs, particularly in elementary school cafeterias, with statements such as "eating meat builds strong muscles." This is because meat sources are considered to contain the highest sources of protein. Unfortunately, meats also contain considerable quantities of hidden fat. Other complete protein sources include dairy products, eggs, fish, and fowl.

Although the need for protein in the United States is grossly exaggerated, the proper amount of amino acids is indeed crucial. For example, some individuals on weight-loss programs, particularly fasting programs, do not consume enough protein. This can be injurious to their health. If the body does not take in the proper amount of amino acids and grams of protein per day, then it will take the protein from its own muscles. Yes, the body will find a way to produce protein. Unfortunately, it does not distinguish skeletal muscle from heart muscle. Therefore, overzealous fasting and dieting may lead to deterioration of the heart muscle, making a person susceptible to arrhythmias and perhaps even sudden death events. In our hospital weight-loss program, for example, we were particularly careful to maintain the minimal daily protein requirement for each individual. We frequently performed electrocardiograms on these participants to ensure a proper functioning of the heart.

We all need a basic minimum of protein. We need to keep ourselves in a "positive nitrogen balance." If the body results in a negative nitrogen balance, we lose protein from our own muscles. Therefore, it is important to select foods that are good sources of protein. Proteins may come from animal sources such a meat, fish, eggs, milk, but also from grains, vegetables, and fruits. Most of us now know that animal protein such as fish, turkey, and white meat chicken offer complete proteins and are lower in fat than red meats. Eggs contain protein and no fat, but do have high quantities of cholesterol. One egg contains 225 mg of cholesterol which for all practical purposes, is almost the maximum daily requirement as well. The American Heart Association recommends that most people should limit their cholesterol intake to less than 300 mg per day. Most overweight individuals should keep their meat and egg consumption to a minimum. Vegetable sources of protein, though highly desirable, are often deficient in one or more of the essential amino acids. Thus, vegetarians may need to supplement their diets with dairy products or combine other foods to make complete proteins. Excellent sources of vegetable proteins as well as carbohydrates include beans, peas, grains, and lentils, to mention a few.

Carbohydrates make up the the most calories in our foods and should be the major source of nutrients in our diet. They are the primary energy storage molecules found in most living organisms. Carbohydrates come from the plant kingdom. The edible portion of plants is called starch. The walls of most young plants are frequently made up of cellulose and starch containing many sugar molecules linked together. These are called polysaccharides, groups of complex sugars that are found in most of the complex carbohydrates or "starchy foods" in our diets such as peas, beans, potatoes, and corn. Disaccharides consist of two sugar molecules with the familiar names being sucrose (table sugar), maltose (malt sugar), and lactose (milk sugar). Monosaccharides are the simple sugars such as glucose and fructose, and contain only one sugar molecule.

Complex carbohydrates are the predominant feature of a healthy diet. It is important to remember that complex carbohydrates should make up at least 65 to 70 percent of our caloric intake. The American Heart Association recommends at least 50 percent of calories from complex carbohydrates. However, I prefer more calories from complex carbohydrates and less calories from fats. Complex carbohydrates cannot be absorbed quickly into the blood stream, though, unless they are broken down by the digestive process. Once they are digested, the breakdown products from polysaccharides are commonly referred to as glucose. Fructose, a monosaccharide, is found naturally in fruit and honey and is easily converted to glucose. Sucrose (table sugar), which eventually breaks down into glucose, makes up approximately 25 percent of the total carbohydrates we eat and occurs naturally in most carbohydrates, especially in beet or cane sugar and maple syrup.

The primary function of carbohydrates is to provide energy for the body. If there is a positive balance of carbohydrates, the glucose may be stored as glycogen in the liver. Our body needs this glucose to maintain its normal function. While the liver can break down glycogen in situations where glucose is needed but not consumed, it is best to consume carbohydrates on a daily basis to provide a continual energy source.

GUESS HOW MUCH SUGAR YOU EAT?

Simple carbohydrates are most often found in sweet foods such as pastries, cakes, and cookies, which are usually made with refined sugar, particularly cane sugar. The problem with eating large quantities of sucrose is that it contains calories but no vitamins, minerals, or fiber. Simply stated, although such sugar provides energy, it really has no positive effects except satisfying our craving for sweets. *Sugar will increase calories and will cause weight gain.* Such simple carbohydrates should be kept to a minimum as they add nothing to the body but calories. One of our goals in carbohydrate awareness is to increase your consumption of nutrient-dense foods and decrease your consumption of calorie-dense foods. Most Americans are unaware that three-fourths of all the sugar we eat comes in processed foods. Although some of us still continue to use a little white sugar in our coffee, tea, or on our cereal, the amount of "hidden" sugar in breads, soft drinks, candies, cakes, and donuts is extremely high. *The average American, for example, consumes approximately 100 pounds of sugar per year!*

Consuming simple carbohydrates also causes a metabolic stress to the body. Simple sugars require less digestion. So when ingested, the sugar molecules enter the vascular system more quickly than other nutrients, thus causing stress on the pancreas, resulting in high insulin releases. Such high amounts of insulin are required to metabolize the sugar. This may result in metabolic swings in our body, alternating between periods of high blood sugar and then low blood sugar. These periods are experienced as mood swings manifesting both high and low energy. After a high insulin surge, for example, low blood sugar may result causing fatigue and light-headedness. This frequently occurs after the "coffee break." During the coffee break we may consume coffee with simple white sugar added and perhaps a donut. Such an increase in simple sugar results in an increase in insulin. After the initial surge of insulin, the blood sugar usually drops. For this reason, we may be hungry again not long after our coffee break. This sets up a vicious cycle resulting in the need of stimulation, such as taking another cup of coffee and donut followed by a very high calorie lunch. Caffeine is yet another ugly player in this game which we will discuss in a subsequent analysis.

Since glucose is the brain's only food, the brain utilizes a considerable portion of the glucose in the body. Unlike other muscles and organs, the brain can burn neither fat nor protein, except in situations of a very prolonged fast. Therefore, low blood sugar, indeed, affects the brain. Symptoms of fatiguability, light-headedness, and dizziness easily occur.

The advantage of eating more complex carbohydrates is not only for their additional vitamin, mineral, and fiber content, but also in time required for metabolism. The more unrefined the carbohydrate, the slower the release of glucose into the blood stream. The more refined the sugar, the more quickly glucose is placed into the blood stream, resulting in higher surges of insulin and later possible symptoms of hypoglycemia. Thus, simple carbohydrates should be kept to a minimum at all times, whereas complex carbohydrates should make up not only the majority of our total carbohydrate intake but also the majority of our diet. Diets high in complex carbohydrates include fruits, vegetables, and grains, thus providing large amounts of fiber as well as nutrients. This is a key factor in any discussion on nutrition and health.

CHAPTER 5

FIBER: THE GOOD

This chapter could save your life.

Most doctors would agree that a diet high in fiber results in a reduced risk of developing many chronic diseases. The importance of fiber in human health has been demonstrated by large population studies. African people on high-fiber diets have a very low incidence of coronary artery disease, colon-rectal cancer, diverticulosis, gallbladder disease, or constipation. The African Bantu population, for example, has an average cholesterol of 90 to 100. In this culture, coronary artery disease is practically nonexistent. Primitive cultures tend to rely on wheat, corn, rice, and grain.

These complex carbohydrates that we mentioned in the previous analysis are exceedingly more productive for the body than the refined carbohydrates and simple sugars that are found in processed Westernized foods. The harvesting of meat for slaughter is also a relatively recent addition to civilization. Was man ever meant to eat meat? If we compare the teeth of man to the teeth of a dog or a cat, we can easily distinguish the absence of carnivorous incisors in man's mouth. Carnivorous animals, those relying on flesh in the diet, in general do not succumb to coronary artery disease. They have genetic protection because they were intended to eat meat.

Civilized man, on the other hand, has a diet composed of meats and fats and yet has a vascular system that is not accustomed to such abuse. Such a drastic change in Western man's diet has been associated with a multitude of diseases including dental caries, diverticular disease, large bowel cancer, hiatal hernia, coronary heart disease, diabetes, gallstones, and obesity. Over the last two centuries there has been a profound change in man's diet. Although hunter/gatherers did consume animal protein, they were dependent upon seasonal migratory habits of herds. Therefore, their meat intake was limited. The most drastic changes in Western man's diet have included an increase in meat, fat, and sugar, and a decrease in coarse carbohydrates and dietary fiber (**Table 1**).

TABLE 1

Changes in Food

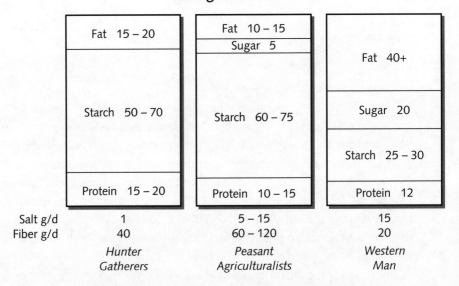

	Hunter Gatherers	Peasant Agriculturalists	Western Man
	Fat 15 – 20	Fat 10 – 15	Fat 40+
		Sugar 5	
	Starch 50 – 70	Starch 60 – 75	Sugar 20
			Starch 25 – 30
	Protein 15 – 20	Protein 10 – 15	Protein 12
Salt g/d	1	5 – 15	15
Fiber g/d	40	60 – 120	20

From *Medical Applications of Clinical Nutrition* Copyright © 1983 by Keats Publishing, Inc. Published by Keats Publishing, Inc. New Canaan, CT. Used with permission.

Dietary fiber is the part of the plant food that our systems cannot digest and when ingested, passes through the small intestine unchanged. How many of us, for example, have changed a baby's diaper only to find the outer shells of corn kernels are still intact even though their nutrients had been absorbed? The absorbable portion of corn is starch. The insoluble or undigested fiber increases the speed of transit through the intestines. Insoluble fiber includes cellulose, heavy cellulose, and lignin – the supportive skeleton of plants and the fiber found in most fruits and vegetables. Soluble fiber, on the other hand, includes pectins, gums, and mucilages. These entities make up the intracellular cement of plants and have several positive effects on the body that promote health and help prevent various disease states. Soluble fibers form a gel-like material that inhibits cholesterol and LDL absorption. Gums are effective in reducing blood glucose levels and in addition may prohibit cholesterol absorption. Pectins also have been shown to reduce blood lipids as well. *The familiar phrase "an apple a day keeps the doctor away," is well spoken.* Apples are a good source of pectin.

Most complex carbohydrates contain both types of fiber. The predominant type of fiber depends upon the plant species. Wheat bran, for example, contains more insoluble fiber than soluable or viscous fiber. Oat bran, rich in gums, is considered a better source of viscous fiber. Insoluble fiber is also found in cabbage, broccoli, turnips, brussels sprouts, kidney beans, green beans, chick peas, nuts, cereals, breads made from whole grain wheat, rye, oats, barley, and corn. Fruits, especially the skins, are also an excellent source of insoluble fiber. Soluble fiber is found in specific fruits such as strawberries, peaches, apple pulp, and citrus. Berries and seeds of fruit are especially rich in soluble fiber.

FIBER HELPS PREVENT COLON CANCER

The physiological effects of dietary fiber occur from our first mouthful of food. High-fiber foods are "chewy." Chewing stimulates the flow of saliva and secretion of gastric juices. Such prolonged chewing also gives the brain a message of satiety. For example, if we chew coarse brown rice, or a high-fiber cookie for that matter, the increased time it takes for swallowing creates a conversation between the brain and the stomach. Since it may take several seconds to perhaps several minutes to ingest such high-fiber foods, the stomach has more time to register the feeling of fullness. Such high-fiber meals fill the stomach and provide a feeling of fullness particularly when ingested with generous quantities of water. The combination of water and fiber swell the stomach, satisfying hunger quickly. Soluble fiber also delays gastric emptying.

In the small intestine, insoluble fiber reduces the rate of digestion and nutrient absorption. In the large intestine, dietary fiber, particularly the insoluble form, increases the bulk of stools. Fiber has a water holding capacity that prevents water from being absorbed through the colonic mucosa in the large intestine. This helps prevent dry, hard stools, thereby alleviating constipation. In general, cereal grains containing cellulose and fruits and vegetables containing pectin serve as excellent bulk forming natural laxatives. Fiber, as we previously stated, increases fecal transit rate. *Therefore, it may protect us against colon cancer because of its laxative effect.* The quicker the waste is eliminated, the less time is allowed for carcinogens to be formed by bacteria and possible chemical reactions in the bowel.

Statistics from population studies all over the world suggest that a high-fiber diet is protective while a high-fat diet may enhance the risk of colon cancer. Consider the United States and Finland, two countries that have a high incidence of colon cancer. Both of these populations consume high-fat diets, but colon cancer mortality is significantly lower among the Finns who consume a much greater amount of cereal fiber than the Americans. The problem with the "normal" American diet is that it contains too much fat and not enough fiber. The average American consumes between 11 and 17 grams of fiber. The National Cancer Institute recommends at least a daily consumption of 20 to 30 grams of fiber (**Table 2**).

TABLE 2

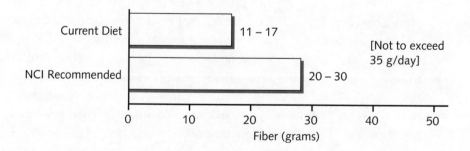

Recommended Daily Fiber Intake Compared with Current Intake

Reprinted with permission from ©1990 Health Learning Systems, Inc.

I recommend 30 with 35 being the maximum. This is essentially twice the daily intake of a typical American, estimated at 11 grams for women and 17 for men. *Diet, therefore, is an important contributing factor in colon cancer. It has also been estimated that 35 percent of all cancers in the country are caused by improper diet.* Since colon cancer, in general, is more prevalent in obese persons, a high-fiber diet is especially essential for this group.

As fiber gives bulk to food without providing additional energy, fiber-rich foods offer excellent advantages to the obese population. It is also an important consideration in the diabetic population as well. A diet rich in complex carbohydrates including fiber may improve blood sugar by offering a large continuous supply of energy rather than short bursts, thus perhaps reducing the amount of medication required. The American Diabetic Association suggests that patients who have diabetes mellitus should double their fiber intake. It is important to consider that diets rich in fiber also contain less fat and cholesterol and fewer calories. This too is as beneficial as weight reduction is in treating the diabetic condition.

FIBER HELPS THE HEART

These implications are also exceedingly important when one considers the causes of coronary heart disease. In experimental studies, soluble fiber sources (pectin, guar gum, barley, and oat bran) have been shown to reduce blood cholesterol levels when taken in generous amounts. We have all heard of the cholesterol lowering effects of oats and oat bran. As little as two ounces of oat bran per day can reduce your cholesterol from seven to 10 percent. Actually, any oat product, i.e., oat bran, oatmeal, or even Cheerios for that matter, are effective as cholesterol-lowering agents. A small percentage of the population may be resistent in this regard.

Recently, the media has questioned the validity of oat bran, indicating that larger amounts may be needed to lower one's cholesterol. While this may be true, if oat bran is supplemented with other fiber-rich foods it creates an additive or synergistic effect on the body. I personally favor oat bran and oat products, particularly since they are excellent sources of soluble fiber and in clinical studies have demonstrated definite reduction in LDL cholesterols in many people.

Wheat bran, on the other hand, has a less significant effect on cholesterol because it is an insoluble fiber. Wheat bran, however, is considered by some to be the best bran to eat in reducing the risk of colon cancer. As previously mentioned, it helps to sweep away the possible cancer producing substances from the intestines by enhancing fecal bulk and increasing transit rate. Insoluble fiber acts in several ways to reduce blood cholesterol as well. This type of fiber may prevent the absorption of many chemicals, particularly the bile acids, into the intestines. Bile acids are necessary to form cholesterol in the body.

Thus, if there is a restriction of bile acids because of altered absorption and greater secretion, this results in the continuous drain of the natural body stores of cholesterol. By the same token cholesterol may also be trapped by fiber and lost through the stools rather than be absorbed. Pharmaceutical companies in this country have created substances that act in a similar way, but doesn't it just make sense to increase our intake of dietary fiber? Why take a synthetic drug if we don't have to? In addition, fiber-rich complex carbohydrates serve as a good alternative to foods high in fat, as recently published in the **New England Journal of Medicine;** people who eat more fiber foods eat less fat foods. Therefore, it makes sense to increase the fiber in our diet. Western diets are too high in fats, sugar, and salt, and too low in fiber and starch. To put it simply, *Americans need to eat more like the inhabitants of some of the undeveloped countries in the world.*

Increasing our starch and fiber, reducing our sugar and salt, and omitting as much fat as possible should not present any major difficulties. We do not deprive ourselves if we consume fiber. The risk/benefit ratio is exceedingly high. Although there are some potential adverse effects such as bloating, cramps, or flatulence, these symptoms are only fleeting and will disappear when our own intestinal flora adjust to the change in the nutritional environment. One drawback of fiber-rich foods may be that they inhibit the absorption of minerals, including calcium and iron. But vitamin and mineral supplementation, or the increased consumption of yellow and green vegetables and fruits, will help in the replenishment of such minerals. Other rare potential hazards of fiber include the remote possibility of obstruction of the GI tract, particularly occurring in individuals who have undergone surgical procedures for peptic ulcer, stomach cancer, or ulcerative colitis.

These individuals should consult their physicians when utilizing high-fiber diets.

Remember, however, most diseases are helped or prevented by fiber, including not only diabetes, diverticulitis, and colon cancer, as we mentioned, but also coronary heart disease. The risk/benefit ratio of fiber is overwhelming on the side of benefit. By increasing the amount of fiber in diet, we can gradually enhance the quality of our health, feel better, and help to prevent many of the illnesses of modern man (**Table 3**). In addition to the Roger Buffaloe cookie, which contains seven grams of fiber, I have prepared a list of other foods that, when combined, also have favorable fiber content (**Table 4**).

TABLE 3

REPORTED HEALTH BENEFITS OF DIETARY FIBER

- Laxation
- Reduction of serum cholesterol levels in hypercholesterolemic patients
- Displacement of fat, saturated fat, and cholesterol from the diet
- Improvement of glycemic control among patients with type II diabetes mellitus
- Treatment and prevention of diverticulosis
- Reduction of colon cancer risk

Reprinted with permission from ©1990, Health Learning Systems, Inc.

TABLE 4

QUICK AND EASY
FAST FIBER COMBINATIONS

FOOD COMBINATIONS	GRAMS OF DIETARY FIBER	TOTAL COMBINED FIBER
1 raw carrot with	2.4	7.3 grams
½ cup raisins	4.9	
1 pear with	5.0	7.1 grams
2 graham crackers	2.1	
3 cups popcorn with	3.0	6.7 grams
1 cup dried figs	3.7	
½ cup cantelope with	2.7	6.6 grams
3 dried prunes	3.9	
½ cup blueberries with	2.5	5.8 grams
⅔ cup Shredded Wheat	3.3	
1 baked potato with	3.7	5.7 grams
½ cup apple sauce	2.0	
¾ cup oatmeal with	2.8	5.7 grams
1 mango	2.9	
⅔ cup Raisin Bran with	3.6	5.3 grams
½ cup apple sauce	1.7	
½ cup brown rice with	2.4	5.3 grams
1 apple	2.9	
½ cup corn (cooked) with	3.9	5.3 grams
1 slice whole-wheat bread	1.4	

CHAPTER 6

CHOLESTEROL: The Bad

Cholesterol is a topic of much conversation these days. The public is so frequently inundated by media and advertising regarding the health hazards of high cholesterol that this topic is of interest to both the healthy and the unhealthy alike. Almost every patient I have in my practice wants to know his or her cholesterol count, the young and the old, those with and without heart disease. But what is cholesterol? And why is there so much conversation regarding it?

Cholesterol is a fatty, wax-like substance, both manufactured by the body and taken in through foods. It is needed in the production of hormones, cells, and bile salts. (For example, cholesterol is a source of the adrenal steroid hormone [cortisone] as well as the sex hormones.) Since our liver manufactures cholesterol, it would reserve enough to support the daily functioning of the body, even if we did not eat any cholesterol at all. Without cholesterol, our cells could not function. We need cholesterol for membrane synthesis, particularly in the stabilization of our cells. In small amounts, therefore, cholesterol is vital to our health and survival. But whenever a person eats beyond his energy requirements, a surplus amount of cholesterol accumulates in the blood. In addition, the liver feeds on the saturated fat to produce even more cholesterol. It is this gradual buildup of white fat and cholesterol that increases the risk of atherosclerosis, which consequently increases the risk of coronary heart disease and stroke, as well as peripheral vascular disease. When too much cholesterol gets into the blood, it may become sticky or sequestered in vessel walls, resulting in a gradual hardening and narrowing of the arteries. This hardening of the arteries is known as atherosclerosis. This artery-clogging action of cholesterol creates plaque in the vascular channels and heightens the risk of cardiac illness. There are many large population studies which indicate that as one's cholesterol rises, one's risk of coronary artery disease also rises.

LOWER YOUR CHOLESTEROL AND LIVE!

Consider the Japanese whose diet mainly consists of rice, fish, and sea vegetables. This culture has the lowest incidence of coronary heart disease in the world. The American diet, on the other hand, consists of considerable quantities of saturated fat found in meats, oils, nuts, and dairy products. The Americans have one of the highest rates of coronary heart disease in the world. The well known Framingham Study, for example, clearly demonstrated that there is a direct relationship between coronary heart disease and a typical American diet. This study began in 1948, and utilized more than 5,000 subjects from Framingham, Massachusetts. The subjects were analyzed in regard to health habits such as diet, smoking, high blood pressure, etc. The results indicate that the higher the cholesterol intake, the greater the probability in developing heart disease. Currently, approximately one in four Americans has a high blood cholesterol. *The good news, however, is that if your blood cholesterol is high, you can reduce your risk of heart disease by simply lowering it.*

A landmark study (Coronary Primary Prevention Trial) by the National Heart, Lung, and Blood Institute showed the benefit from lowering cholesterol is considerable. In this trial, each one percent reduction in blood cholesterol was associated with a two percent reduction in coronary heart disease risk. Thus, participants who reduced their cholesterol by 25 percent, reduced their risk of heart attack by almost one-half. Other studies have also demonstrated that *lowering cholesterol levels actually can reverse the buildup of blockages in coronary vessels, resulting in a regression of atherosclerosis.* Since the medical literature is so overwhelmingly supportive in the direct relationship between cholesterol and coronary heart disease, every reputable physician should counsel his or her patients about the potential hazards of cholesterol. Physicians do frequently recommend that patients know their cholesterol numbers and take a more active role in healing themselves, particularly through dietary choices.

As a matter of fact, I have found that patients nowadays have become so aware and so knowledgeable about cholesterol that they not only want to know their total numbers, but also ask questions regarding HDL and LDL, lipoproteins that carry cholesterol in the blood. The blood is like sea water and cholesterol is a fat. Since water and fat do not mix, cholesterol is carried in the blood in combination with a protein, referred to as high-density lipoproteins (HDL), and low-density lipoproteins (LDL). HDL cholesterol, commonly called "good" cholesterol, is considered to be a type of cholesterol scavenger in the body. HDL picks up cholesterol from blood vessels and transports them back to the liver. LDL, on the other hand, infiltrates the blood vessel walls, thus increasing the risk of "plaque" buildup in the vessels. If the plaque buildup occurs in the coronary vessels, this could render an individual susceptible to heart disease. LDL is a noxious substance by itself and, especially when combined with the toxic effects of cigarette smoking or the membrane-tearing effects of high blood pressure, it results in a gradual inflammatory process that invades the blood vessel wall, causing a buildup or a proliferation of the vessel, resulting in gradual closure. Thus, the higher the LDL, the more one is at risk for heart disease. Conversely, the higher the HDL, the more protection one has from heart disease.

Cardiologists frequently not only look at total cholesterol, but also at the cholesterol fractions of LDL and HDL. Individuals who are at the most serious risk for developing coronary heart disease include those people with a low HDL and a high LDL. So, doesn't it make sense to increase your HDL and lower your LDL? One way to increase HDL is by *losing weight,* as studies prove they have an inverse relationship. *Vigorous exercise* is another effective way to raise the HDL. Effective ways of lowering LDL also include weight loss, as well as *reduction of fat in the diet,* utilization of more *dietary fiber,* and *cessation of cigarette smoking.* Cigarette smoking is indeed a major cardiovascular risk factor, not only because of the toxic effects of tar and nicotine, but also because cigarette smoking enhances the effect LDL has on the vascular wall. In a recent European study, smoking was found to increase the total cholesterol and cause a reduction in the HDL, particularly in women.

EMOTIONS AFFECT CHOLESTEROL

In addition to smoking and diet, there are many other factors known to affect cholesterol. For example, *emotions* are a major consideration. Calming touch has been shown to actually lower blood cholesterol while stress increases it. Yes, it is true that excessive stress and tension can affect the regulation of cholesterol in your body, regardless of the intake through diet. Scientific studies have shown that accountants during tax season who are under severe deadlines to perform have considerable elevations in their blood cholesterol during the months of January through April. Following the tax season deadline of April 15, their cholesterol levels would then fall. Conversely, animal models have demonstrated that rabbits who received preferential care from their handlers actually had lower cholesterol deposits than rabbits who did not receive such cuddling. Therefore, cholesterol is not only influenced by genetics and diet, but also by one's emotional and psychological well-being.

Levels of blood cholesterol can vary considerably among different individuals. How do you know if your cholesterol is too high? Recently the National Heart, Lung, and Blood Institute panel of experts have advised standard guidelines for doctors and their patients (**Table 5**). Individuals with total cholesterols below 200 mg per deciliter appear to have a more favorable profile than individuals with cholesterols greater than 240. Patients at serious risk for coronary heart disease also include those with HDL levels less than 25 and LDL fractions greater than 160. LDL levels below 130 mg per deciliter are considered desirable. HDL greater than 65 mg per deciliter are also considered protective. (Thus, most doctors and patients would agree that it is necessary not only to know your total cholesterol, but also to know the fractions of LDL and HDL.)

THE CASE OF DR. JOSEPH GUARDINO

Dr. Guardino, a medical internist from Manchester, Connecticut, had a known cholesterol problem, with his total serum cholesterol calculated at 230 with an HDL of 48, and an LDL greater than 160. This type of profile, according to the National Cholesterol Education Program, is considered high risk for coronary artery disease. He also weighed approximately 180 pounds and was 25 pounds overweight. In addition, his genetic history included a malignant family history of heart disease; that is, his father, also a physician, at age 50 had a heart attack and unfortunately succumbed to heart disease ten years later.

Dr. Guardino took a serious look at his lifestyle habits, weight, and hypercholesterolemia. He knew of the work I was doing in high-fiber/low-fat therapies for weight reduction. He was also especially interested in the Buffaloe cookie because of its simplicity. He then proceeded to go on a high-fiber/low-fat diet. He ate two cookies a day in combination with generous quantities of water. He frequently would use one cookie as a snack and an additional cookie for the lunchtime meal. He was careful about omitting fat in his diet and was conscious of consuming greater than 30 grams of fiber per day. Over a period of three months, he lost approximately 25 pounds on his high-fiber/low-fat diet. He was astonished to find that his cholesterol went from 230 to 154. He was encouraged, to say the least. After his first cholesterol was drawn, however, he did not believe the results. He continued to persist on his high-fiber/low-fat regimen and had a second cholesterol determination done a few weeks after the first. Although his total cholesterol increased to 180, however, his HDL (or protective cholesterol) also increased to 67 which is extremely favorable. This cholesterol profile virtually contains no risk at all.

Now, approximately nine months later, the saga of Dr. Guardino continues. He has managed to keep the weight off. He still continues to consume two cookies a day and he has managed to stay on his high-fiber/low-fat *Lose to Win* program. Although the case is anecdotal, the profound biochemical effects in this physician's cholesterol profile are noteworthy. The increase in HDL, the decrease in LDL and total cholesterol were probably modified by both a combination of weight reduction and a change in dietary awareness.

TABLE 5

NATIONAL CHOLESTEROL EDUCATION PROGRAM

BLOOD CHOLESTEROL LEVEL	RECOMMENDED ACTION
Greater than 240 High	Refer to physician
Between 200-239 Borderline High	Refer to physician
Less than 200 Desirable	Repeat in 5 years

Although HDL can be modified by exercise and weight reduction, most doctors would agree that the reduction of saturated fat is the most important way to lower the LDL in your diet. Saturated fatty acids increase plasma cholesterol levels. It is a simple fact that cholesterol in the blood increases as a result of taking not only cholesterol in the diet, but also saturated fats. Approximately fifteen percent of total calories in the typical American diet comes from saturated fatty acids, which is one reason Americans have such high serum cholesterol levels. Saturated fatty acids that have the greatest impact on raising cholesterol include lauric acid, myristic acid, and palmitic acid. Other nutrients, particularly linoleic acid (polyunsaturated fatty acid) and oleic acid (a monounsaturated fatty acid), may reduce LDL concentrations and its bad effects.

While there is some controversy about the mechanism of LDL reduction, it is undisputed that using polyunsaturated and monounsaturated fats, such as olive oil, instead of saturated fats, such as butter, will reduce LDL levels. When the body takes in saturated fatty acids, the liver transforms them into blood cholesterol. Butter, for example, has little cholesterol, but has 99 percent fat, so when it is ingested the liver converts a portion of it to cholesterol.

CHOLESTEROL CULPRITS

Another way in which our diet choices can increase our cholesterol levels is simply through an increased intake of total calories. Obesity, commonly associated with an increased caloric intake, for example, increases serum cholesterol simply on the basis of more ingested calories. Obesity can also result in lowering the HDL (good cholesterol). Weight loss, on the other hand, will help to reduce the LDL levels.

A major recommendation for lowering cholesterol is to reduce the intake of total calories. Again, this means reducing our total fat intake in grams. Reducing the level of saturated fatty acids and replacing them with monounsaturated fatty acids and small quantities of polyunsaturated fatty acids is also recommended. Recently, however, it was suggested that one should utilize more polyunsaturated fatty acids in the diet, but investigations have indicated that such an increase in polyunsaturated fatty acids may actually result in lowering of the HDL. This is an undesirable effect that we wish to avoid. A better alternative is to use more monounsaturated fats, such as *olive oil* and *canola oil*. A more detailed description of polyunsaturated and monounsaturated fats will be given in the subsequent analysis on fatty acids. For now, I ask you to focus your attention on the cholesterol effects of saturated fat.

Saturated fats are found predominantly in foods of animal origin such as meats, organs, butter, cream, cheese, and most dairy products. Very high amounts of saturated fats are also found in chicken fat, beef fat, and particularly in organ meats such as heart, kidney, and sweetbreads. Other saturated fats include coconut oil and palm oil, frequently used by manufacturers in processed foods and packaged baked goods. *Coconut oil is approximately 99 percent saturated fat,* actually containing higher percentages of saturated fat than butter or meat. It is important to recognize that these oils are used in nondairy creamers as well as commercially prepared whipped creams and vegetable shortenings used to prolong shelf life and prevent rancidity. A good rule of thumb is to *limit our intake of commercially prepared baked goods, meats, saturated fats and oils.*

We should also lessen the intake of dairy products and eggs. Did you know that *one of the most cholesterol-producing items in the American diet comes from milk?* Milk fat found in dairy products including milk, butter, cheese, cream, and ice cream, not only contains high amounts of cholesterol, but also saturated fats. It is essential for weight loss and lowering cholesterol levels to reduce these items in the diet. For example, whole milk contains approximately 50 percent of total calories from fat. It is advisable to gradually shift to two percent milk, which is preferable to whole milk but still contains about 36 percent of calories from fat, down to one percent fat milk, which contains about 18 percent of calories from fat. Skim milk is the most preferred. Skim milk and one percent milk really do not contain excessive amounts of fat and they are also rich in protein and calcium, so it is not necessary to totally eliminate dairy from the diet. It is strongly recommended, however, that individuals with high serum cholesterol and those who want to lose weight use either very low fat or skim milk whenever possible. Butter, cream, cheese, and ice cream should be eaten infrequently and only in small quantities as they contain both high levels of saturated fat and cholesterol. Low-fat substitutes are also available for all of these items.

Eggs are another culprit. Each egg yolk contains approximately 225 mg of cholesterol. Since the recommended intake of cholesterol is less than 300 mg per day, it is suggested that eggs be cut to a minimum. Egg whites, on the other hand, contain no cholesterol and are also an excellent source of protein. Egg substitutes contain no cholesterol, but some researchers say that they contain saturated fats. Since eggs contain considerable quantities of protein and particularly important minerals such as magnesium and sulfur, I am not recommending that we discard eggs completely from our diet. To consider eggs, we simply need to be more prudent and aware of other components in our diet. For example, the average American consumes approximately 600 mg of cholesterol per day as opposed to the recommended 300 mg. Unfortunately, the egg industry has taken a beating in this regard. The "all American" breakfast of two eggs, bacon or sausage, buttered toast, and sweetened coffee has approximately 700 mg of cholesterol. Since two eggs contain approximately 450 mg of cholesterol, it is no wonder that the egg industry and the Heart Association are at variance with one another.

In Montauk, on the tip of Long Island, I met a surf fisherman named Bob. He was a successful contractor only in his mid-forties who recently sought advice from his physician for a typical chest discomfort. During the evaluation, his cholesterol was 275 (undesirable) and his triglycerides, another measure of fat in the blood, were 900, which is extremely undesirable. He told me that for 30 years his early morning breakfast was two eggs, bacon *and* sausage, with toast and coffee. After seeing his physician, who recommended a prudent diet, his cholesterol came down to 180 and his triglycerides to 260. Incidentally, after six months of choosing the proper foods, he lost 12 pounds! With such metabolic improvements, his risk of coronary disease is considerably lower. Whole eggs are an excellent choice for nutrition. They are a poor choice for cholesterol.

SOME HEALTHY SUGGESTIONS

Organ meats have the highest cholesterol of all known tissues. Three ounces of sweetbreads, for example, contain approximately 2,600 mg of cholesterol! This is one item that should be absolutely forbidden to any health-conscious individual. *Other items that I recommend be forbidden to people who want to stay healthy include processed meats such as bacon, salami, sausage, hot dogs, and bologna.* These items should be avoided because of their high content of saturated fatty acids and calories, not to mention harmful nitrites and sodium levels. *Most hamburgers are 70 percent fat.* All of these meats mentioned above are also high in cholesterol. Preferable meat choices would include chicken and turkey (without skin), although dark meat chicken contains similar amounts of cholesterol to beef. White meat turkey, on the other hand, has lower amounts of cholesterol and saturated fatty acids than chicken and is recommended as a meat substitute. Wild goose is another good alternative.

Although trimming the fat from meats and removing chicken skins does reduce the amount of fat and cholesterol, frequently the ingested cholesterol goes unnoticed, as in marbled meats. Such marbling in the meat contains high quantities of fat, later converted to cholesterol and, therefore, should be avoided. *If you insist on red meat, however, the best cuts are London broil or top round steak,* particularly if used in hamburgers. If you ask the butcher to trim all the excess fat and grind the meat for hamburgers, they will have approximately four to five grams of fat per serving as opposed to 20 grams found in chuck burgers. For my cardiology patients who like red meat, I frequently recommend a recipe (included in this book) for an eye of round. Again, this is what nutritional awareness is all about.

Another alternative to meat is fish. Cardiologists usually recommend two to three helpings of fish per week to their patients. Fish is rich in the Omega-3 fatty acids that are beneficial to the cardiac patient. Omega-3 type fatty acids, or fish oils, are not found in significant quantities in most foods other than small amounts in soy beans, walnut oils, and flax linseed oil. Most researchers agree that *Omega-3 fatty acids have the favorable affect of making the blood less sticky.* Therefore, this decreases the likelihood of blood clots forming. Population studies, particularly from the Netherlands, Japan, and the Greenland Eskimos, seem to indicate that diets rich in fish products lower the incidence of coronary disease. A typical Eskimo diet, for example, has about 40 percent fat calories coming from whale, seal, and fish.

Despite this high percent of dietary fat, the incidence of coronary heart disease in Eskimo men is extremely low. Like the Japanese, who also ingest large quantities of fish, the Eskimos are protected from the epidemic of coronary heart disease that plague the Western societies. Perhaps the cod liver oil that your mother used to give you as a young child really was good for you! Fish oil is the most preferred of all the oils. Although it makes sense to avoid as much oil as possible, fish oil, olive oil, and canola oil, followed by safflower oil and sunflower oil, are the most preferred. My own recommendation would be to permit fish oil and use olive oil in moderate amounts.

Shellfish is considered by many nutritionists to be taboo because of its high content of cholesterol. In reality, however, most shellfish do have acceptable levels of cholesterol with the exception of squid. Squid contains approximately 250 mg of cholesterol per 100 grams. Crab, lobster, oysters, and clams have lower levels of cholesterol. It is true that shellfish do contain more cholesterol by weight than poultry and even some red meats, but it is lower in saturated fats. As a clinical cardiologist, keeping this data in mind, I would not restrict the amount of shellfish in the diet. It would be prudent, however, to use less squid and shellfish and more of the other types of seafood.

We also need to remember that the medical literature does support Omega-3 fatty acids from fish as a positive factor on platelet function, making blood less sticky, thus reducing the risk of coronary events. Alterations in platelet function may have an effect on one's overall mortality. This was recently shown in a two year study in male survivors of myocardial infarction in which a moderate intake of fatty fish and fish oil decreased total mortality by 29 percent. While this effect occurred without any reduction in serum cholesterol levels (in this study), Omega-3 fatty acids in cold-water fish or shellfish can cause slight lowering in lipids and small decreases in LDL cholesterol without affecting HDL cholesterol.

A word of caution, however, about fish, shellfish, and fish oils: Fish caught in coastal waters may be contaminated with pesticides, heavy metals, and PCB's. As a striped bass and bluefish fisherman, I can attest to my concern about this problem. It is true that fish can be easily contaminated, as heavy metals and PCB's may reside in their fat. The recommendation here is to *cut out as much of the dark meat from the fish as possible, as this is the fatty part.* It usually occurs in the center of the fish and toward the tail. With careful dissection, many of the pollutants found in this heavily oiled section can be eliminated. Taking vitamins, minerals, and other antioxidant agents may also be helpful and are antagonistic to such pollutants. *Therefore, I do go on record as recommending Omega-3 fatty acids.*

The grain and vegetable oil sources of Omega-3 fatty acids already mentioned are also beneficial. Pumpkin seeds and soy beans supply small amounts of Omega-3 fatty acids as well. Cholesterol is not found in these oils nor in grains, fruits, and most vegetables, but olives and avocados are particularly high in total saturated fat and should be limited. Coconut, coconut oil and palm oil should also be avoided for this reason. Most processed foods or preserved foods contain coconut oil and/or palm oil, so be sure to read labels! Processed foods reporting palm or coconut oil should be absolutely avoided. In the next chapter we will discuss the issue of fat, both the hazards and potential benefits, of most oils.

CHAPTER 7

FAT: THE ISSUE

German singer, Ernestine Schumann-Heink, struggled through the orchestra pit in a cramped Detroit concert hall, knocking over music racks with every step. "Sideways, madam," the conductor urged in alarm. "Sideways!"

"Mein Gott!" cried the singer in reply. "I haff no sideways!"

On another occasion, Enrico Caruso saw her seated in a restaurant with a very large steak on her plate. "Stina," he said, "surely you are not going to eat that alone?"

"Of course not alone," she laughed, "mit potatoes!"

Fat constitutes almost half of the total calorie consumption of Western cultures. As stated previously, it comes in various forms. Fats are the most calorie-dense food we eat. In addition to providing our bodies with considerable energy for our muscle needs, fat also provides insulation against cold and protects us from injury. In our food, fat improves the taste and frequently makes us feel full. Biochemically, fat is a chemical combination of carbon, hydrogen, and oxygen atoms. Saturated fats contain single carbon chains with hydrogen atoms attached. Monounsaturated fats have fewer hydrogen atoms than saturated fats, and polyunsaturated fats have still fewer hydrogen atoms attached to the carbons. It is this hydrogenation (adding hydrogen atoms) that makes the oils more saturated. Hydrogenation also yields an oil with a more solid consistency at room temperature and a longer shelf life. So the more hydrogenated an oil, the more saturated it is, thus the more harmful it is.

As you know from the analysis in the previous chapter, saturated fats usually come from animal products, with the exception of coconut and palm oil, and their high intake has been linked to an increased cholesterol and thus a greater risk of heart disease. Unsaturated or polyunsaturated fats are liquid at room temperature and most come from plant sources. These compounds usually contain double bonds as opposed to a single bond found in saturated fatty acids (**Table 6**). Examples of polyunsaturated fats include sunflower oil, corn oil, and grape seed oil. Monounsaturated fats are composed of a fatty acid chain with only one double bond. An example here would be the oleic acid found in olive oil. Thus, if the fatty chain has more than one double bond it is called a polyunsaturated fat (PUFA). Recent research indicates that monosaturated fats such as olive and canola oil are the least threatening to the cardiovascular system. However, we need to be very conscientious of the fact that all oils are 100 percent fat and all oils, therefore, contain some saturated fat. Although olive oil and canola oil contain mostly unsaturated fats, they do contain small quantities of saturated fat and will raise cholesterol levels. Remember that one tablespoon of any oil contains 14 grams of total fat. I recommend that you keep the consumption of oils to a minimum, but if you need to choose an oil, it would be advisable to *use either olive oil or canola oil.* My own particular preference, possibly fostered by my Italian heritage, includes *cold pressed extra virgin olive oil.* I use this type of olive oil in my salads and in most of my cooking.

TABLE 6

Representation of Chemical Bonds in
Saturated, Monounsaturated, Polyunsaturated Fats

SATURATED	MONOUNSATURATED	POLYUNSATURATED
H H H H H H	H H H H H H	H H H H H
-Ċ-Ċ-Ċ-Ċ-Ċ-Ċ-	-Ċ-Ċ-Ċ-Ċ=Ċ-Ċ-	-Ċ=Ċ-Ċ=Ċ-Ċ-
H H H H H H	H H H H	H

Olive oil is an interesting entity in itself. Several years ago while doing research for a presentation in Brussels on the cultural and international aspects of heart disease, I learned that the island of Crete had an insignificant incidence of heart disease when compared to several other countries in Western Europe. In fact, the data indicated that not one person on the island of Crete died of a myocardial infarction over a 10 year period. However, the cholesterol for an average inhabitant of Crete is over 200. This presented somewhat of a paradox for me. The author indicated that it must have been the sunny climate and lack of stress that resulted in the lower incidence of heart disease. I felt that the lack of emotional stress and tremendous family camaraderie and support was a major factor in the low incidence of heart disease. I have since realized, however, the residents of Crete eat tremendous quantities of olive oil. As olive oil has been shown to preserve good HDL and lower LDL, perhaps these effects were significant despite the average cholesterols being over 200. It is best to use extra virgin olive oil because it is cold-pressed and because it is of the highest quality, being pressed only once.

When substituted for saturated fatty acids in the diet, olive oil and other MUFA'S such as canola and almond oil lower LDL levels. They do not appear, however, to reduce HDL. This is a favorable point of information. PUFA's will lower LDL when substituted for saturated fatty acids. However, large intakes of PUFA's are also associated with lowering of HDL. This is not favorable for the cardiovascular system. In addition, animal studies have also demonstrated that high intakes of PUFA's may promote tumor development after pretreatment with chemical carcinogens. This is just one of the distinct advantages of monounsaturated fats over the polyunsaturated fats.

For example, olive oil (a MUFA) has been reported to have blood-thinning properties and contain antioxidants that may help prevent early cell death. Although some of us prefer the taste of polyunsaturated fats, clinical research favors monounsaturated fats for optimal health. While the beneficial Omega-3 is a polyunsaturated fat found in fish, its effect on platelets is such a positive factor on the cardiovascular system that I recommend it as well. Canola oil is a MUFA that comes from grapeseed and it has a lighter taste than olive oil. The only fatty acid that is essential is linoleic acid, the polyunsaturated fat found in corn oil and safflower oil, among other vegetable oils. Since the body cannot make its own supply, we need to take this in the diet. But this type of essential fatty acid should only comprise about two percent of our daily calories and it can also be obtained from oatmeal.

HAVE FUN READING LABELS

Keeping this data in mind, you ought to read labels carefully when you shop. But food labels sometimes don't tell us "the whole truth." For example, *some labels may state no cholesterol, but that does not necessarily mean they won't contain saturated fat, which, when ingested, will be transformed to cholesterol.* Additionally, the word "hydrogenated fat" may be used as a euphemism for the highly saturated palm oil and coconut oil. So be aware and beware! *The best thing to do when reading labels is to look at the content of saturated fat, polyunsaturated fat, and monounsaturated fat* (**Table 7**).

TABLE 7

COMMONLY USED FATS AND OILS

TYPE OF FAT	SATURATED	MONOUNSATURATED	POLYUNSATURATED
Almond oil	1.3 (grams)	9.1 (grams)	3.6 (grams)
Beef fat	7.1	6.0	0.5
Butter	9.0	4.1	0.6
Canola oil	0.8	8.4	4.4
Chicken fat	4.2	6.4	3.0
Coconut oil	11.7	0.8	0.2
Corn oil	1.7	3.4	7.9
Cottonseed oil	3.6	2.6	6.9
Fresh Flax	1.3	2.2	10.5
Grape seed oil	1.6	2.4	9.9
Lard	5.6	6.4	1.6
Margerine	2	5	4
Mayonnaise	2	3	7
Olive oil	1.9	9.8	1.2
Peanut oil	2.6	6.2	4.1
Pumpkinseed oil	1.2	4.8	8.0
Safflower oil	1.3	1.7	10.0
Sesame oil	1.8	6.4	5.7
Soy oil	2.0	3.1	7.8
Sunflower	1.4	2.8	8.7
Walnut oil	2.2	3.9	7.8

AVOID HIGHEST SATURATED FAT	SUBSTITUTE HIGHEST MONOUNSATURATED	SUBSTITUTE HIGHEST POLY W/OMEGA-3
Coconut oil	Olive	Flax
Butter	Almond	
Beef fat	Canola	
Lard		

It is important to organize your shopping around low-fat, low-cholesterol concepts. Reading labels can also be fun. When reading labels, it is interesting to try to figure out the percentage of calories from fat. For example, if we are on a 2,000 calorie diet, the recommended fat intake is approximately 20 percent. Twenty percent of 2,000 is 400 calories. Four-hundred calories equals approximately 44 grams of fat. Thus, this should be our total fat intake for the day. (The American Heart Association Diet is more lenient with 30 percent calories from fat. I prefer 20 percent.) Of this total fat intake, only 10 percent of the fat intake should come from saturated fat. This means that only four to five grams of fat should come from saturated fats.

In addition to organizing your menu around fats, it is also important to keep tabs on the fiber content. Remember that by increasing the fiber content and reducing the fat content, weight loss may be considerable (**Table 8**). If you are going to *Lose to Win*, you need to know your daily intake of fat. Remember we are not counting total calories but only the grams of fat (**Table 9**). In my own particular situation, I try to take in less than 25 grams of fat per day. Again, this is the equivalent of a one-quarter pound hamburger with cheese found in many of the fast food restaurants. Keeping the intake of grams of fat to a respectable level will not only reduce total body fat, but will also reduce caloric intake.

In our previous discussions we mentioned that excess calories are predominantly stored in the body as fat; you're familiar with this type of fat that is around the waistline, thighs and backs of our arms. Cardiologists refer to this as "triglycerides in the body," but in simple terms this is our body fat. Body fat can be determined by anthropometric measurements using calipers. Accumulation of body fat is a simple mechanism. We either eat too much or we exercise too little.

TABLE 8

HIGH-FIBER/LOW-FAT FOOD

Food	Serving Size	Fiber	Fat (g)	Calories
Health Valley Chili	5 ounces	12.2	3	160
All Bran	⅓ cup	8.6	1	70
Multigrain Pancake mix (Arrowhead Mills)	3 pancakes	8.0	2	290
Prunes	5 large	7.9	Trace	115
Roger Buffaloe Cookie (Oatmeal Raisin)	2 oz.	7.0	2	192
Old Wessex Irish Style Oatmeal	⅓ cup	7.0	2	110
Chickpeas	½ cup	6.2	Trace	115
40% Bran	¾ cup	6.0	1	95
Kidney Beans	½ cup	5.8	Trace	110
Pinto Beans	½ cup	5.3	Trace	115
Slit Peas	½ cup	5.1	Trace	115
Pear	1 pear	5.0	1	110
Raisins	½ cup	4.9	Trace	220
Broccoli	1 spear	4.5	Trace	55
Lima Beans	½ cup	4.4	Trace	105
Peas, green	½ cup	4.1	Trace	65

TABLE 9

MAXIMUM FAT INTAKE

Most of us are unaware of how many calories we should eat, much less how many grams of fat we should intake. The following chart is a helpful index regarding your daily caloric needs as well as the maximum total fat allowance. For the purposes of this chart, your caloric needs are determined by your activity. For example, if you are very active, multiply your weight in pounds by the number 16. If you are moderately active, multiply by 15. If you are inactive, multiply by 14, and if you are sedentary, multiply by 12. For someone like myself, weighing approximately 150 pounds and being moderately active, I would need 2,250 calories of which my maximum fat intake would not exceed 50 grams. Being a cardiologist, however, I am aware of the hazards of fat intake and, therefore, probably eat less than 25 grams of fat per day, which is approximately 10 percent of total daily calories from fat. In the *LOSE TO WIN* philosophy, if you can keep your fat intake to less than 20 percent per day, as well as increase the fiber intake, you will gradually lose weight. The following table offers examples of the maximum fat intake per day. To figure out your caloric intake, use the formula as suggested.

MAXIMUM TOTAL FAT INTAKE
MODERATELY ACTIVE – MALE & FEMALE

IDEAL BODY WEIGHT	CALORIES	FAT (G) PER DAY
120 (lbs.)	1,800	40
130	1,950	43
140	2,100	47
150	2,250	50
160	2,400	53
170	2,550	57
180	2,700	60
190	2,850	63
200	3,000	67
210	3,150	70
220	3,300	73
230	3,450	77
240	3,600	80
250	3,750	83

SINK OR SWIM

In our passive exercise study of women at the New England Heart Center, we determined the amount of fat in several areas of the body. In our study we concluded that exercise in combination with a high-fiber/low-fat diet actually reduced body fat. Significant reductions in body fat were noted, particularly in the suprailiac (waist) and triceps (back of upper arms) areas. Although fat does have its functions, most Americans have too much body fat. There is some disagreement but it is safe to say that 15 to 20 percent of body fat for men and 20 to 25 percent body fat for women is considered the maximum range for a healthy person. One can be slightly out of this range and still be healthy, but it is my belief that less body fat is more acceptable. We should strive to keep our body fat to a minimum.

We also need to know that as we get older our body fat increases. This is why the older we get the easier it is to float in water. I remember when I was a collegiate wrestler I had less than 10 percent body fat. I was also taking scuba diving lessons at the time. During my certification for scuba diving, it was apparent to everyone in the class that I did not need lead weights to get me to the bottom. I indeed had negative buoyancy. I sank like a rock! Neither could I float as other people could. I really thought there was something wrong with me. I thought I perhaps had heavy bones or lead in my pants. What I really had was less body fat than all the others, and since fat is lighter than muscle, they floated. Being able to float is a direct response to having body fat. I was too dense to float! Thus, one consolation to getting older is being able to float in the ocean!

Through my training as a cardiologist, I have been able to keep my weight down almost to my college wrestling level. This nutritional awareness has been a long-term process for me. Gradually, I have been able to reduce the saturated fat in my diet, but only to a point where I still don't feel deprived. For example, most of my diet includes vegetables, grains, and pastas. Although I used to be a terrific meat eater, I have reduced my intake of meat, only having red meat on rare occasions and poultry approximately one to two times a month. But there is also another reason why I avoid fat in the diet. I really believe our planet is in danger. Numerous chemicals and pollutants that affect the earth are being absorbed first in roots and vegetables and later in the animals that consume them. Just as PCB's and mercury are stored in fish fat cells, pesticides and other chemical pollutants are stored in animal fat cells. As you can see from the graph, pesticides and pollutants increase as the fat chain increases (**Table 10**). Pesticides and chemical pollutants are another reason why we need to consider reducing the fat in our diet. This is an area of intense investigation that you need to be aware of for your overall and physical health.

Fighting cancer is another reason why we need to decrease the fat in our diet. There are several studies that show the casual relationship between fat intake and the occurrence of cancer. Population studies as well as studies in animals show convincing evidence that *an increase in the intake of total fat increases cancer particularly of the breast and colon.* Researchers from the Harvard School of Public Health found that men with the lowest fat intake had half the rate of precancerous colon polyps as men with the highest fat intake. The Harvard study also demonstrated the impact of fiber in that the high-fiber group (greater than 34 grams a day) had only one-third as many polyps as the group with the lowest fiber intake (less than 17 grams a day). In addition to cancer and cardiovascular disease, obesity, diabetes and gout are also associated with high-fat intake. If the weight of all these negative effects of fat consumption does not serve as a "noteworthy factor" to make some dietary changes, I don't know what would. Maimonides, in 1198, was indeed correct when he stated the simple fact, "fat is bad."

TABLE 10

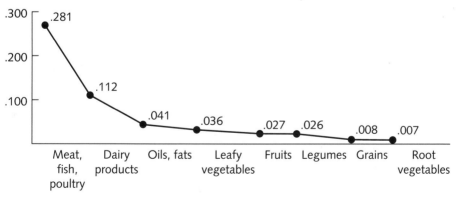

Pesticides and Food Groups

Source: *Runner's World*

CHAPTER 8

SALT, WATER, ALCOHOL, AND CAFFEINE

Are you a drinker? I hope so.

The human body is mostly made up of water. The blood, for all practical purposes, is similar to seawater. Water is involved in almost every body process including digestion, absorption, and excretion. Water helps maintain the proper body temperature and is essential for carrying waste material. Since water is continuously lost through excretion of urine, elimination, sweating, and breathing, it is important to replenish the proper amount of water each day. Most researchers agree that drinking at least eight glasses of water a day is necessary for good health. And water is also germane to weight loss. Studies have shown that a decrease in water consumption will cause an increase in fat deposits while an increase in water can actually reduce the amount of fat in the body.

The mechanism is simple. If the kidneys cannot function properly due to dehydration, some of that responsibility has to be taken up by the liver. Since the liver metabolizes stored fat for energy, it cannot work at full capacity if the kidney is compromised. Therefore, the liver metabolizes less fat, and more fat then remains in the body, resulting in weight gain.

Water is an extremely important catalyst in weight loss. For example, in the Optifast program each participant had to drink large quantities of water continuously. If water was not consumed adequately, dehydration would occur and weakness and lethargy would result. When utilizing Roger Buffaloe's high-fiber cookies, at least two glasses of water or other fluid needs to be taken with each cookie in order to fully maximize the benefit of the seven ounces of fiber. Water also causes the fiber to expand in the stomach and increases the feeling of satiety. The best way to give your body water is to replenish it. Since water is a major factor in fat metabolism, it makes sense for the overweight person to drink as much water as possible. The health implications of drinking plenty of water are numerous to say the least. In addition to helping rid the body of toxins, water can help relieve constipation as well. When the body gets too little water or too much salt, or if the patient is given too much diuretic, the body takes water from its internal sources. The colon is one such source. The result is constipation.

WATER TRICKS

Drinking enough water is not only essential to weight loss, but is also essential to good health. In medical school, for example, I trained with one of the top kidney experts in the United States. He was one of the original investigators of kidney dialysis. When we used to make rounds in the hospital wards *my professor would never pass a water fountain without drinking.* By watching him I learned a lot. He continuously drank water each day to give his kidneys the nurturing they needed. If that was good enough for a professor of nephrology, it was certainly good enough for me. I tried to remind myself as much as possible about the medical consequences of deficient water intake. In summary, *we need to drink at least eight eight-ounce glasses of water every day. This is about two quarts of fluid. During weight loss, we should drink at least one glass of water during each meal and a glass at least one hour prior to the meal.*

As previously stated, too much salt depletes our natural stores of water. Excess sodium in the diet causes unnecessary fluid retention in the tissues, even edema, and depletion in other parts of the body such as the colon and upper gastrointestinal tract. In order to flush ourselves of salt we need to drink more water. Too much common table salt (sodium chloride) is harmful to our bodies in many ways. In higher concentrations it disturbs mineral balance in the body. Too much salt in our diets can cause fluid buildup, thus creating an increase in pressure. This can lead to high blood pressure and possibly heart disease.

The National Cholesterol Education Program (NCEP) recommends a sodium intake of less than three grams per day. Excessive salt intake has been incriminated in disease not only in urbanized societies but also in primitive societies as well. Natives in the Caribbean who cook their foods in seawater, for example, had much higher levels of blood pressure than those who cooked in fresh water. *In order to get rid of extra body salt we need to drink more water.* As water is forced through the kidneys, it takes away the excess sodium.

Unfortunately, salt does not only come from the salt shaker. Processed foods make up approximately 50 percent of the average American diet and these foods often contain a considerable amount of hidden sodium. Again, we need to read labels. For example, some of the commercially prepared soups contain almost a gram of sodium per can and a fast food hamburger may also contain at least one gram of sodium. A large kosher dill pickle contains greater than one gram of sodium. An over-consumption of processed foods with little dietary awareness leads us to be vulnerable to excess sodium in our diets. For example, we need to be aware that additional sodium is often added to bread products. Salt in this country is considered to be an excellent preservative.

Since sodium occurs naturally in most foods as well as water, there is no danger of our bodies not getting enough. You really don't need any additional sodium chloride. Salt is not a food; salt has no nutritional value. The only time I would favor utilizing salt is in individuals who are losing a lot of sodium chloride through excessive work and perspiration. Elderly patients suffering from low blood pressure who do not have any heart muscle disease may also be permitted to use salt. Under these circumstances the best way to get salt into the body would be in the form of natural fruits and vegetables. Celery and sea vegetables, for example, contain natural quantities of sodium chloride in its organic form.

LAST CALL FOR ALCOHOL

Alcohol is another source of empty calories providing no vitamins, minerals, or other essential nutriments. This is certainly one type of beverage that should not be utilized in anyone trying to undergo weight reduction. Alcohol just adds calories to the diet. It is really not a food, but rather a drug. Alcohol may be considered a poison. It causes metabolic damage to the body and depresses the immunological system. As a clinical cardiologist I can attest to the amount of heart disease that alcohol causes. I have seen hundreds of patients, for example, with no previous known history of heart disease come into my office with "heart muscle disease." The most common etiology of such heart muscle disease, in the absence of other factors such as coronary artery disease, viral illnesses, or valvular heart disease, is alcohol-induced cardiomyopathy.

Studies on alcohol are too numerous to count. But one particular study shows that at least two ounces of alcohol per day can cause deterioration of the heart muscle over a short period of time. This was seen in one study in which a group of volunteers drank two ounces of Vodka per day and the control group drank water. At the end of the experiment, the ones who took alcohol had heart muscle deterioration on microscopic analysis. In addition, alcohol can damage almost any cell in the body. The heart, the brain, and the liver are perhaps the most vulnerable. Much of my medical internship and residency included treating alcoholics. The amount of disease entities common to alcoholics is incredible: Pneumonia, liver disease, arthritis, eating disorders, delerium and dementia, and nerve and muscle disease are common to the alcoholic. The emotional destruction that alcohol causes is almost as profound as the physical destruction.

Another important fact to consider about alcohol is its effects on insomnia. Alcohol is probably the leading cause of insomnia. While alcohol does not induce ideal sleep, in some individuals it may cause the body to be anesthetized, seeming as though in a deep sleep. The sleep pattern, however, is not a good one. After ingesting alcohol and particularly after eating sweets, perhaps in a dessert after a nice dinner, many people have difficulty falling asleep because of the vasodilating effects of alcohol and the rapid heart rate that follows.

One of the most common things I see in my office is alcohol-induced cardiac arrhythmia. The patients come in with all different scenarios about skipped heart beats, irregular heart beats, and rapid heart beats, much of which has its origins in taking alcohol. Other causes may be emotional distress, which is frequently compounded by the patient's use of alcohol as a remedy. Overall, my recommendation on hard alcohol is to try to avoid it.

Wine, on the other hand, has been used as a healing remedy for centuries. While it is not a good idea to drink it every day, wine contains polyphenols which are agents that kill viruses and bacteria. Polyphenols, like some vitamins, have antioxidant capabilities or the ability to tie up free oxygen radicals that cause destruction to cells. Since it contains antioxidant properties, it perhaps has some beneficial anti-cancer properties, as well. Some investigators have also touted the use of an evaporated wine residue to be used as a remedy in treating cold sores and Herpes Simplex infections. The low alcohol content in wine may offer yet another advantage in healing. Recent investigations have supported the hypothesis that light alcohol consumption may actually reduce the risk of coronary heart disease, perhaps by favorably influencing HDL and blood clotting mechanisms. Wine, however, is alcohol and like caffeine it needs to be used in moderation.

A WORD TO THE WISE ABOUT CAFFEINE

Caffeinated beverages such as coffee were once highly regarded as a drug used by physicians in Western Europe. In 1859, it was utilized as a respiratory treatment and written up in the medical journals as the prescription of choice for bronchial asthma. The pharmacological properties of caffeine are similar to the xanthines, a group of compounds that stimulates the central nervous system and the heart, as well as relax smooth muscles (especially the bronchial tubes) and empower the brain. Caffeine also acts as a diuretic, resulting in increased blood flow to the kidney, thereby allowing more water to be excreted. Drinking a cup of coffee and getting stuck in a traffic jam can have some undesirable consequences.

The average American citizen consumes approximately two to five cups of coffee a day, which contain between 200 and 300 mg of caffeine. Decaffeinated coffee does contain caffeine but in insignificant quantities. Caffeine is also found in chocolate, tea, and cocoa. A cup of tea usually contains less than half the amount of caffeine as a cup of coffee (Table 11).

Excess caffeine intake has been noted in young children who drink colas. The symptoms of irritability, hyperactivity, and insomnia are frequently due to excess quantities taken into the body. In my own clinical practice, I have seen scores of patients with problems related to caffeine intake. For example, my most recent case (occurring in September of

1991), involved a young 25 year old male with a history of a psychiatric disorder. Since his psychiatrist prescribed tranquilizers to control his mood, he was referred to me for cardiological evaluation because of an exceedingly high heart rate, frequently greater than 120, and a blood pressure as high as 220/120.

An in-depth medical history on this individual, however, disclosed that he was drinking ten cups of coffee per day. He was also drinking considerable quantities of cola beverages. This individual suffered not from a "drug-induced" heartbeat problem, but from *caffeinism*. This is a condition where the heart rate and the blood pressure increase and the patient feels very irritable and hyperactive. Patients will frequently complain of an erratic heartbeat, skipping of the heart, and fluttering. Frequently they will also have insomnia. The treatment of this condition is simple, one needs simply to reduce and perhaps cut out all caffeine intake. I have counseled several patients on similar conditions of this type. Many patients have come to me with cardiac arrhythmias who simply were ingesting too much caffeine.

TABLE 11

AVERAGE CAFFEINE CONTENT OF SELECTED ITEMS (MG)

BEVERAGES

SOFT DRINKS (12 OZ SERVING)	CAFFEINE (MG)
Cherry cola, Slice (Diet or Regular)	48.0
Cola-Cola (Diet or Regular)	46.0
Cola (decaffeinated)	0.18
Mellow Yellow	53.0
Mountain Dew	54.0
Pepper type	37.0
Pepsi Cola, Diet	36.0
Pepsi Cola, Regular	38.0

COFFEE SERVING SIZE	CAFFEINE (MG)
Brewed, Regular 6 oz.	103.0
Brewed, Decaf 6 oz.	3.0
Instant, Reg 1 rounded teaspoon	57.0
Instant, Decaf 1 rounded teaspoon	2.0

TEA HOT/COLD SERVING SIZE	CAFFEINE (MG)
Brewed Commercial 5 oz.	20-50
Brewed Imported 5 oz.	25-80
Instant 5 oz.	10-20
Iced Tea 12 oz.	70
Crystal light 8 oz.	11

MILK SERVING SIZE	CAFFEINE (MG)
Chocolate Flavor Dry Mix with milk 2-3 teaspoons	8
Chocolate Syrup in whole milk 2 tablespoons	6
Cocoa/Hot Chocolate with water 4 teaspooons	6

CANDY

CHOCOLATE SERVING SIZE	CAFFEINE (MG)
German Sweet (Bakers) 1 oz.	8
Semi-sweet (Bakers) 1 oz.	13
Milk-Chocolate (Cadbury) 1 oz.	15

OVER-THE-COUNTER DRUGS	CAFFEINE (MG)
Anacin	32
Excedrin	65
No Doz	100

Caffeinated beverages, especially coffee, have also been known to enhance gastric acid secretion, and aggravate ulcers. Every physician knows that when a patient is suffering from excess acid production or abdominal discomfort to instruct them to avoid caffeine, alcohol, nicotine, and aspirin, as these are the four most common harmful chemical compounds that affect the gastrointestinal tract. Caffeine, like nicotine and alcohol, is considered a drug and, therefore, we must weigh the potential benefits versus the hazards. Some physicians believe coffee is harmful and should be avoided altogether. Others, myself included, feel it is okay in small quantities. The benefit for one individual may be increased mental mood, alertness, and concentration. An undesirable effect, however, could be lethargy and fatigue as a result of low blood sugar occurring an hour after consuming the coffee. Although caffeine has indeed been used to treat bronchial asthma, excess caffeine may render the heartbeat irritable and cause an increase in blood pressure. I know, for example, that during my days as an athlete, and particularly during my days as a medical student, I relied on caffeine to keep me mentally alert and physically sharp. Coffee is definitely considered a "pick me up."

On the other hand, we can really poison our bodies with too much caffeine. Please understand: caffeine is indeed a drug with considerable side effects. *I would recommend consuming no more than one to two cups of coffee per day and none after 3:00 p.m.* Decaffeinated beverages may be consumed in moderation. In summary, caffeine, like alcohol, needs to be considered carefully. Although deprivation does not need to occur with these beverages, caution needs to be exercised when using them. Remember, *the best beverage is water* and definitely a major player in the *Lose to Win* philosophy.

CHAPTER 9

EXERCISE

Consistent involvement in aerobic exercise has been repeatedly shown to be associated with multiple health benefits, including alleviation of occupational stress and reducing psychological strain. In weight loss, exercise is crucial. In addition to the negative energy balance resulting from exercise, many individuals feel that it also reduces their appetite. During a strenuous work-out the body burns carbohydrates into sugar, and a higher blood sugar in itself will assuage the appetite. However, we really don't have to exercise strenuously for weight loss or optimal health. This is a myth. Many cardiologists, myself included, do not recommend jogging or running. Estimates indicate that between 45 to 60 percent of the almost 20 million runners in the United States injured each year are hurt seriously enough to require an adjustment of their running habits.

We have all heard of healthy people having accidents while jogging. Such occurrences may include strained muscles, tendonitis, back injuries, knee sprains, and even the rare occurrence of the dissection of the aorta and sudden death. Excessive running has been reported as causing delayed menstruation and amenorrhea in women. Jogging in polluted environments on roadways with excessive exhaust fumes is frankly unhealthy, as is jogging in very hot or cold weather which may result in heat exhaustion, frostbite, or even dog-bite.

The benefits of exercise, however, are considerable. Exercise has been shown to control several of the cardiovascular risk factors including obesity, high blood pressure, diabetes, and elevated blood lipids. Dynamic exercise with the secondary effects of conditioning may result in a lower heart rate and blood pressure. In cardiovascular rehabilitation we exercise people after heart attack and bypass surgery to improve physical endurance. Once an individual improves his physical conditioning, this may result in the heart utilizing oxygen more efficiently and thereby increasing the amount of exercise that can be done before developing chest pain. *Angina* is a term doctors frequently refer to as a situation of coronary insufficiency when blood flow to the heart muscle is decreased and there is insufficient oxygen supply. This may present as a heart cramp, pressure, or burning in the chest.

Exercise can reduce body fat and increase muscle mass. An important and beneficial metabolic result of exercise is an increase in serum HDL levels. High endurance and aerobic exercise such as cross country skiing are excellent in increasing HDL. Other biochemical considerations of exercise include a reduction in the stickiness of blood, which may prevent the blood clots that cause heart attacks. Other favorable effects on insulin and glucose metabolism occur. In women, exercise also protects against osteoporosis.

Perhaps the greatest benefit of exercise is the reduction of emotional stress. Exercise has been known to assuage the driven Type-A behavior pattern and is an alternative way to utilize the peripheral muscles instead of our precious heart muscle under situations of high stress and arousal. In this way, dynamic exercise can interrupt a chronic state of visceral-vascular readiness and assuage the overactive nervous and cardiovascular systems. *So enough about the benefits, how much is needed and how should we go about it?*

MAY I HAVE THIS DANCE?

Although there is considerable debate about how much exercise is necessary to promote optimum physical and emotional well-being, it is my feeling that *any amount of activity is better than none.* We showed this in a passive versus active exercise study at The New England Heart Center that was published in the ***Journal of Cardiopulmonary Rehabilitation.*** In approximately 94 women who were placed in various groups, i.e. control, walking, and passive exercise, any activity proved beneficial when matched against controls. Even the passive exercise toning tables appeared to be as beneficial as walking to overall health and reports of well-being. Although the walkers had better cardiovascular fitness, the women who performed on the toning tables also had the same favorable metabolic and physical improvements in their health and well-being. When measured with calipers, they both lost the same amount of millimeters of fat as well.

The study was extremely provocative because it showed that even simple walking or passive exercise promotes improvement in metabolic, physiological, and psychological profiles. Therefore, it really is not necessary for optimal health to get involved in strenuous forms of exercise such as high-impact aerobics, running, or racing for that matter. *The term "no pain, no gain" is totally untrue.* Any activity, active or passive, will have some beneficial effect.

In my opinion, walking and dancing are the best forms of exercise, as simple everyday activities that can indeed make a difference in your overall cardiovascular health. Just walking the dog is an excellent activity that is as good for you as it is the dog. Walking is a form of aerobic exercise. Other types of aerobic exercise that strengthen the heart and improve circulation include cycling, swimming, skiing, and some calisthenics. Isometric exercises, on the other hand, such as heavy weightlifting, and resistance exercises, including waterskiing, do not improve the conditioning of the heart. Rather, these types of exercise may increase strength and perhaps add extra muscle or provide additional bulk to the body. It is aerobic exercises that cause us to breath deeply, expanding the chest and thereby providing more oxygen to the heart and the rest of the body.

The reason why athletes have a lower heart rate than sedentary people is because the heart pumps more blood with each heart- beat. Since the average heart rate is close to 72 beats per minute, conditioning usually has occurred when the resting heart rate comes down to approximately 60 beats per minute. In some of the professional athletes I have treated, it is not uncommon to see the heart beat in the 40 to 50 range. The heart is a muscle, and like our biceps and calves, can be gradually strengthened. If the heart beats rapidly and wildly under conditions of simple aerobics, this is a sign of poor conditioning or oversympathetic arousal. In the conditioned person, the heart rate will remain steady only gradually increasing with aerobic activity. The fit individual may even combat stress and emotional trauma better than a physically unfit person. After all, one of the greatest advantages of exercise is a release of stress and tension in the body.

If you wish to consider a more advanced exercise program than walking the dog, I recommend that you see your physician prior to beginning exercise. If you are over 40, your physician may recommend an exercise stress test to determine the possibility of any cardiovascular risk. For those who wish to exercise and raise their pulse rate to greater than 120 beats per minute, an exercise evaluation is an excellent screening tool for weeding out individuals at risk. If you do not wish to involve yourself in a formal exercise program, you may wish to perform daily passive exercise.

NOT THE REMOTE CONTROL!

Passive exercise is simply accomplished by doing your normal daily activities, but instead of using machinery, you are using your own legs. Passive exercises include such things as walking to the train station or bus station, parking the farthest away from the entrance of your place of employment, using the stairs instead of the elevators, taking a walk perhaps during lunch time, and most importantly, *throwing away the remote television control.* For those who wish to involve themselves in a more formal program, the following are a few tips to make your fitness and exercise program more enjoyable:

1. Find a convenient time and place to exercise. (This may be before breakfast, during lunch, or after work.)

2. Try to avoid the heat of the day or the nocturnal hours.

3. Set a definite goal such as walking one mile or cycling 20 minutes three times a week.

4. If you miss an exercise session, make an agreement with yourself that you will make it up at a later time.

5. After you have lost two pounds or a half inch on your waistline, reward yourself by treating yourself to something such as a movie, a haircut, a manicure, or a sports event.

6. Keep your exercise program enjoyable and varied.

If you feel motivated, and I hope you do, and wish to engage in more brisk aerobic forms of exercise, you will need to consider a warm-up period of stretching and breathing. The first set of exercises may include the four following maneuvers:

EXERCISE 1

This exercise includes abdominal breathing. Lie on the floor and bend the knees, keeping your feet on the floor. With your eyes closed and your hands over your navel, breathe out naturally and feel the abdomen push against the hands. Again, breathe nasally with a full inspiration and expiration. This form of breathing can be practiced prior to any exercise session or even meditation.

EXERCISE 2

After developing a sense of abdominal breathing, lie on the floor with the pelvis extended and the knees bent. Insert a rolled up blanket in the small of the back and place the feet securely on the floor. You will feel a sensation of stretching in the abdomen that will allow fuller and deeper breathing. This is also a good stretch for the lower back. You may wish to push your buttocks into the floor to accentuate the stretch.

EXERCISE 3

This is a back exercise. Lie down on the floor. Bring your knees to your chest and then swing them to the right and then to the left. This frees up the lower muscles of your back. While keeping your lower back on the floor, swing your knees back to your chest. Gently rock yourself forward and backward several times so you are rocking on your lower back region. Remember not to strain yourself. Repeat this six or seven times and then gradually get up slowly.

EXERCISE 4

For this exercise, place your hands on your hips and bend at the waist, bringing your torso down toward your knees. Bend as far as possible without straining. While keeping your hands on your hips, you may feel a mild stretching in your lower back and then your hamstring muscles at the backs of your calves. Now, come to the upright position. Spread your legs as wide as possible with the toes pointed inward. Now, place your knuckles in the small of your back and lean backward as far as possible while opening up your throat by releasing a sound. This will stretch the muscles in the chest, diaphragm, and neck. Remember again, do not strain yourself. Do this five to ten times.

These exercises will take only about five minutes. They are excellent exercises to stimulate your breathing and provide stretching to the legs, abdomen, chest, and lower lumbosacral spine. After you have done this warm-up you can then choose to exercise as you like. In choosing an exercise, we should consider several aspects: how long, how much, and how often. Now we are getting into the realm of physical fitness that includes guidelines for an exercise prescription. Following are the components:

1. Type of activity
2. Duration of activity
3. Frequency
4. Intensity
5. Progression.

Fitness experts, such as doctors in the American College of Sports Medicine, of which I am a member, have established the following recommendations for the quantity and quality of exercise in order to develop and maintain both body composition and cardiovascular fitness:

TYPE OF ACTIVITY – *Aerobic exercise is preferable for fitness.* Aerobic activity stimulates breathing by using large muscle groups in a continuous and rhythmical form. Such exercises include jogging, running, walking, hiking, dancing, swimming, skating, rowing, cross country skiing, jumping rope, and bicycling.

DURATION OF ACTIVITY – *Fifteen to 60 minutes of continuous or discontinuous aerobic activity* is required for health and fitness. For example, to perform 15 minutes of rope skipping continuously would be difficult. To perform this type of activity for three to five minutes, however, taking a short rest, and then continuing for a total of 20 minutes is manageable and effective. Fast walking can also be performed for a 20 minute stretch. Since walking is not as intense as rope skipping, it does not need to be discontinuous, though both are aerobic.

FREQUENCY – *Three to five times a week* is considered by most sports experts to be an appropriate frequency for exercise.

INTENSITY – The intensity of activity can vary. Most fitness experts are in agreement that *between 70 to 85% of one's predicted maximal heart rate* is a good reliable index of intensity. For example, suppose you had an exercise stress test with your physician, and your maximal heart rate obtained during that evaluation was 150 beats per minutes. If you take 70% of 150, this equals 105. Eighty-five percent of 150 equals 127.5. Therefore, if you exercise in an aerobic activity and wish to enhance your cardiovascular fitness, your exercise target heart rate should be between 105 and 128. Although there are other formulas that have been advocated, this is the easiest way for developing an exercise prescription. For the unfit or overweight individual, this exercise prescription is perhaps the safest, especially when constructed from an exercise treadmill evaluation. In this case, an exercise program should only be utilized with the advice of your physician.

PROGRESSION – In the unfit or overweight individual, little progression or increase is advisable. If, however, you have begun to notice improved fitness and a reduction in weight, you may *increase your total work effort by perhaps 10 percent per month.* However, recommended rates of progression varies with individuals. It is usually best to progress slowly and increase gradually in a spirit of keeping your motivation and interest intact and not torturing yourself. The old motto "exercise till exhaustion," is counterproductive.

THE EXERCISE SESSION

To safely undergo an exercise program, it is necessary to include at least three phases: Warm-up, work-out, and cool-down. Each phase has a particular purpose.

The warm-up phase usually includes the stretching and breathing exercises that we already have mentioned and may last from five to 10 minutes, with the purpose of increasing the body temperature, loosening-up the joints and ligaments, and relieving any undue soreness. A slight elevation in heart rate is also a benefit of the warm-up phase. Generally, *the older or the more obese the person, the longer the warm-up should be.*

The work-out phase usually lasts between 15-60 minutes, with an ideal period of approximately 20 minutes, plus five minutes to warm-up and five minutes to cool down. To improve cardiovascular fitness and body composition, as well as to lose weight, continuous aerobic activities of low to moderate intensity are recommended for positive benefits.

The cool-down phase, which should last from five to 10 minutes, brings back the physiological system toward the resting level at a gradual pace. After a vigorous work-out, our cardiac output may be considerably elevated, perhaps two to three times the resting level for an individual. Thus, it is important to cool-down to permit a gradual readaptation of the body system. One of the best cooling-down exercises, again, is slow walking. After a work-out such as running, jogging, or rope-skipping, a walking cool-down is all that is required. In structured rehabilitative-type exercise programs, such as our hospital's Cardiovascular Rehabilitation Program, the cool-down period usually includes relaxation techniques. For example, after the clients have completed their work-out phase, many of them will walk around the room. After a brief walk, we ask them to lie down and focus on their breathing and then we lead them into a meditation to get them in touch with their bodies and their feelings about their bodies. These procedures are extremely helpful in relieving stress and tension in the cardiovascular system.

So now you know about exercise and how an exercise prescription works. But what are the forms of exercise, and what types of exercise should we do? Let me first begin this discussion with my two favorite types of exercises: Dancing and walking.

DANCING

Dancing is without a doubt the best form of exercise as it incorporates the whole body. The benefits from dancing are enormous. Have you ever seen people put their whole heart into dancing? Their bodies becomes graceful. Their movements are integrated with the music. Their hips, chest, thighs, and arms are coordinated in rhythm with the music. My patients often ask me what types of dancing are best. Any form of dancing will do, whether it is square dancing, ballroom dancing, freestyle, or country western. All have a common denominator: Movement with music.

Dancing is also a great way to get over our inhibitions. One of the best features of dancing is that it gives us permission to use the pelvis, which many of us feel is taboo. The pelvic floor is a major location for the center of energy in our body. By rotating this area, we are able to move the whole body. And dancing can be done alone and at any age.

Have you ever listened to the radio and started to sway to a favorite song? Next time, get up and dance! Don't stop yourself from feeling the music and moving. We put our emotions into dancing. When you see couples close their eyes while dancing slow, do you get a feeling of tranquility and connectedness? Any exercise we put our feelings into, particularly positive feelings, enhances not only the spirit, but also the core of our beings.

By the same token, anyone who has negative energy such as anger or rage, should not, I feel, use strenuous physical exercise to work it out. Instead, I would recommend the releasing emotional exercises described earlier, such as kicking the feet on a bed or verbalizing feelings in a car. Contrary to popular belief, trying to work out anger through exercise could perhaps do a disservice to the body. With rage, we have an increase in adrenalin. Coupled with strenuous exercise, it's like throwing gasoline on a fire – by overcharging the already overstimulated heart, we can overdose on our own hormones. For example, after I resuscitated two victims of sudden death in the emergency room, they both indicated that they had been very angry and were using exercise as a way of discharging their anger. Exercise will not take away anger, but merely burn off some of the excess energy that is associated with it. The way to get rid of anger is to express it in a clean and harmless manner.

WALKING

Walking is also an excellent exercise for all ages. Young and old love to walk. I encourage walking in my older population because of its safety. I rarely have heard of people hurting their legs, ligaments, or knees while walking. Try to take in the surroundings when you walk. And don't worry about the pace. Most exercise enthusiasts believe that we have to walk fast or briskly in order to burn calories. This is not the case. If fact, a mile of walking burns as many calories as a mile of running. Enjoy this activity. Take time for yourself. Move your hips and get into the natural ebb and flow of a rhythmic motion. Feel your body. Feel each step. It can be very enjoyable.

I would recommend a minimum of at least 20 minutes of walking once a day. After you have progressed and feel comfortable about walking one mile, try working up to walking two miles, or better yet, walk 20 minutes twice a day. Again, this should be fun and leisurely. Remember, it costs nothing and you can do it alone. Walking with someone or perhaps in a group will offer an excellent support system.

Many of my patients have commented that walking can sometimes be boring day after day. On the surface, this may be true, so be creative! One can go hiking through the woods or through the mountains for that matter. For example, I am an avid fly fisherman and I frequently need to walk up and down river banks and through the fields to get "where the fish are." Surf fishing is another excellent exercise, moving up and down the beach while casting and reeling and recasting and reeling. I have met numerous surf fishermen well over the age of 60, many of them with their rods in their hands. The anticipation of catching a fish is a feeling for which many fishermen develop an addiction. I know – I have it! Isn't it crazy to get up at daybreak to go fishing? Many a time I wanted to cuddle in the sheets of my bed and not go out in that cold early morning air, but once I started to get ready and anticipate walking and breathing in the fresh ocean spray, my priorities changed. Remember that surf fishing requires walking, and walking next to dancing, is the best form of exercise.

Other ways to incorporate walking into our lives is in the game of golf. Again, this is an activity that is good for both the young and the old. It is so heartwarming to hear of an elderly man score close to his age. I have endorsed golf as an exercise to many of my clients. Although in a cardiovascular sense the amount of exercise is minimal, golf still requires considerable walking. And if you carry your clubs or pull your golf cart, you will even burn up more calories. Although there are many exercise specialists who speak disparagingly of golf, or tennis for that matter, I feel they are excellent activities that are good for both the mind and the body.

Other Exercises

Skiing, both cross-country and downhill, are other types of recreational activities that are excellent forms of exercise. Cross-country skiing gives all the benefits of running without any of the side effects of shin splints, ankle, knee or hip injuries. Instead of pounding on a hard surface, the cross-country skier uses rhythmic movements to gently glide across the snow. Downhill skiing is another form of exercise that again utilizes walking. Although most of us use chairlifts, many downhill skiers do lots of walking. Unfortunately, it usually occurs after losing a ski or retrieving lost equipment!

Other activities I endorse are swimming and cycling. These two non-weight bearing activities are especially good for the overweight or elderly person. Stationary cycling is preferred over outdoor cycling for the elderly or during inclement weather, especially if you live in New England as I do. I frequently tell my patients to cycle for approximately five to 15 minutes. This could even be done with a low-grade tension on the bicycle. If some of my patients get bored, I suggest they listen to the news or turn on the television; some patients even read while stationary cycling. My own recommendation is to let your mind go and just focus on the rhythmic activity of the legs.

Other indoor activities could include climbing stairs or using a rowing machine. As director of our Cardiac Rehabilitation Program, I suggested the rowing machine as one of our preferred forms of exercise. A good rowing machine will exercise almost all the major muscles of the body. When I row, I particularly feel a sensation in my abdomen, arms, and lower back. Rowing also creates a rhythmic activity which I find enjoyable. Rowing to music is a nice way of exercising. Try rowing to classical music with your eyes closed. After a couple of minutes, you may not even realize you are exercising.

A treadmill is another form of exercise I recommend. We also use this piece of equipment in our Cardiac Rehab Center. Participants are asked to walk on a treadmill with a gradual increase in speed and elevation, which they use in conjunction with their exercise prescription. My suggestion here is to just use the treadmill as a walking machine, not another stress test. It is not necessary to increase the speed or raise the elevation to a high degree. For starters, it is best to start with the machine at 1.7 miles an hour with perhaps a five percent grade. If you walk at this pace for three minutes, you are achieving approximately three "mets" of work, a term that cardiologists frequently use to refer to a metabolic equivalent. For example, simply walking at a slow pace is considered to be one to two mets. Walking at a faster pace or up a slight incline is three mets. My recommendation would be to walk at a low level of activity at a low elevation for perhaps 15 to 20 minutes.

Walking on a treadmill is not as good as walking outside because the variety in terrain allows different muscles to be worked. But this can be done as an alternative, particularly when weather conditions are not permitting. Indoor exercise allows you to fit a program to your schedule as time permits, but doesn't have the benefit of support and change of scenery that outdoor exercise programs can offer.

Let me explain what I mean by support. I can remember how an exercise support group was extremely helpful in bringing one of my patients out of a low grade depression. He had recently lost his wife to a sudden heart attack and became very depressed. He, too, was a victim of heart disease, sustaining a massive myocardial infarction only nine months prior to his wife's sudden death. After recovering from his heart attack, he gained a new sense of self only to lose his will to live when his wife died.

Although this was a very fragile man in his 70's, with high-grade coronary artery disease, I advocated an exercise program as a way for him to strengthen his heart and develop a new vital connection. In our Phase III Cardiovascular Rehabilitative Program, he indeed made many such connections and new friendships. In short, he became an exercise enthusiast. He came to the program three times a week and walked and talked with almost everyone. Exercise not only increased the strength of his cardiovascular system, but also gave my patient a new interest in life. The establishment of new vital connections after the loss of a significant other can truly be rewarding and life-sustaining.

Another indoor exercise that I can suggest is *repetitious dynamic light weight-lifting*. This can be done alone at home or with others at a gymnasium. I am recommending it more and more to my patients, even those advancing in age. As we gradually grow older, and particularly after the age of 40, the average man loses his lean muscle mass, which is replaced by fat. Since increasing age is inevitable, it makes sense to exercise isolated muscle groups with light weights. If you prefer to exercise at home, you do not need to go out and purchase barbells, dumbbells, or fancy weightlifting equipment for this exercise. I have even told my patients to try lifting magazines or heavy books after appropriate stretching. Repetitive light weight training is a good way to increase muscle tone, decrease fat, and burn calories. Remember to breath through the lift, exhaling on effort. Always avoid breath holding.

Sit-ups with the knees bent or elevated, perhaps on a bed or chair, is another good activity that can be used in conjunction with weightlifting. Sit-ups are an excellent endeavor in the strengthening of the abdominal muscles. Many of us have had chronic back problems in which simple muscle toning of the abdominal wall will alleviate many of our lower back ailments. Push-ups are also an alternative, but we need to be cautious about utilizing push-ups or sit-ups or even low weights in individuals who are hypertensive or have heart disease, so a stress test may be in order before beginning a formal exercise program. When performing sit-ups, exhale on the effort to lift up, inhale as you slowly lie back down.

Another favorite exercise of mine is *jumping rope.* For this, you will need a good pair of padded athletic shoes and a jump rope that may be purchased in many of the sporting stores. Remember that if you jump rope, *do not jump with both feet at once,* but rather alternate one and then the other. Most of us would agree that five minutes of jumping rope can be quite fatiguing and is equivalent to perhaps 10 to 15 minutes of cycling or rowing! As a wrestler, I used to jump rope for five to 10 minutes as a warm-up exercise prior to our several-minute scrimmages.

In summary, there are many types of exercises we can perform. Aerobic exercise is preferred over isometric exercise. With exercise, we need to be *creative.* To avoid boredom, we may have to switch our daily routines. For example, walking one day, cycling another, and perhaps rollerskating or ice skating on another. If walking is the core in your routine, you can supplement it with recreational activities such as golf and tennis. The point is to try to do some light exercise every day. If you are involved in a cardiovascular fitness program, it is prudent to only exercise three to four times a week at your target heart rate.

HAVE FUN!

Exercise is a cardinal ingredient in weight reduction. Exercise not only increases muscle tone, but also alters the metabolic rate in our bodies; a fit individual will burn more calories than a less fit one. If you are involved in high aerobic activity, I recommend that you get an exercise prescription from your doctor. Remember that exercise can be thought of as a drug or certainly as a therapy that has tremendous benefits, but also some hazards.

You may be wondering why I have not discussed taking your pulse during leisurely exercise activity such as pleasurable walking or dancing. My problem with taking your pulse rates is that it takes us out of our bodies and into our heads. It also takes the fun out of it! You can tell when you're overdoing it. You should not be gasping for breath or dizzy. Listen to your body and nurture it, don't torture it. *The important thing about exercise is to keep it safe and to have fun.*

However, if you are trying to achieve fitness in a high-level aerobic program or following a physician-oriented exercise prescription, you will need to know if the pulse rate is within your recommended guidelines. There are many devices on the market that digitally display the user's heart rate at a glance. I feel these are oftentimes preferable to pulse-taking because they do not take the individual back "into his head" to palpate and compute heart rate. They do allow for a quick check of heart rate to ensure that exercise is within safe guidelines.

Exercise does not need to be a struggle. If you make it fun by choosing an activity you enjoy, you will more easily incorporate it into your daily living program and soon manifest the numerous physiological, psychological, and biochemical benefits that exercise provides.

CHAPTER 10

VITAMINS AND MINERALS

I'd like to share a "Letter to the Editor" I recently wrote to my local newspaper in Connecticut regarding whether or not to take vitamins.

As a physician, father, cook, and recent author who has thoroughly researched the medical literature, I can tell you that although there is no substitute for a balanced diet, the drain of antioxidants on our bodies becomes exhausted. Nowadays many of our soils have become "worn out," water has become polluted, industrial toxicities fill the atmosphere, automobile emissions pollute the environment, heavy metal toxicities are springing up everywhere and nuclear waste dumps are poisoning the depths of the earth. These toxins create an undesirable metabolic stress on the body. One way of protecting our bodies is tying up free radicals with antioxidants. For example, if excessive fat is burned in the body *after* we have just eaten in our favorite fast food restaurant, or if excessive radiation is taken in when we are at the beach on a bright, sunny day, or if toxic fumes are inhaled (driving in traffic on a hot humid day), or if heavy metals are ingested (lead in our drinking water), the body in trying to protect itself, becomes involved in a biochemical war between the invading toxins and our immune system. The by-products of these biochemical reactions may result in toxic wastes accumulating in the body, thereby resulting in hormonal changes which may result in symptoms of allergy, palpitations, nausea, and shortness of breath to mention a few. Such events over the short and long-term may lead to biological changes, diseases, and aging. This is where vitamins and minerals come in.

Although eating fresh fruits and vegetables on a daily basis would help, it is a known fact that transport and storage result in produce losing valuable vitamin content. Take, for example, the comment in the article about eating a fresh orange over vitamins. The question is, how fresh is fresh? And is the orange laced with toxic chemical agents and pesticides? We also need to be aware that many vitamins and minerals are not particulary consumed in the diet. Take Coenzyme Q_{10}, for example, a vital nutrient particularly for the cardiovascular population. Q_{10} is found in abundance in beef heart muscle, pork, mackerel and sardines, but who eats that particular diet? And what about the population on antibiotics, birth control pills, corticosteroids, alcohol, and excessive caffeine? All of the above entities frequently deplete the vitamins and minerals in our body. What about the patient who has undergone coronary artery bypass surgery, who has been placed on a heart-lung machine? It is a known fact that once the blood is circulated through a heart-lung machine, the vitamin, mineral, and coenzyme factors of the blood are destroyed. I could go on and on about why we need vitamin and mineral supplementation in the latter aspect of the twentieth century. Certainly the Japanese do not have a problem with this. Since Co-Q_{10} went on sale in April of 1974, approximately six million Japanese take it every year. If I were writing the article on "To Be or Not To Be Taking Vitamins," I, as a clinical cardiologist, a modified vegetarian who eats very little meat and consumes considerable quantities of grains, fresh fruits and vegetables, and herbs, would continue to *BE* taking vitamin and mineral supplementation and, in addition, continue to recommend them to my family as well as my patients.

As a lay person and particularly as a young doctor, I never held vitamins or minerals in high esteem. After all, I always felt I ate well, and why should I supplement my body when I consumed grains, fresh fruits, and vegetables? Being a doctor, I thought I *knew* what was beneficial. But again, my patients have become my best teachers. Frequently, for example, I would need to prescribe drugs for various conditions. I, like many other doctors, had some pharmacological failures. While sometimes I had to ask myself if my patients were really taking the medications, most truly accepted my advice and followed instructions.

It was only after careful scrutiny and much investigation that I learned many of my patients were not really *absorbing* the medications. Some patients have diminished hydrochloric acid in their stomachs and consequently cannot absorb medicine. Could the same thing happen with foods? If so, how would we know? Through becoming ill? It became increasingly clear to me that whatever agents we put into our bodies may not be absorbed, and even if we were to absorb all the nutrients we eat, is this enough to sustain our bodies optimally in today's environment?

Over the last few years as I continued to read and practice preventive medicine, I gradually began to believe more and more in the healing powers of vitamins and minerals and natural healthy foods. There are subtle changes that may occur in the body which frequently are missed by the individual. In my particular case, I had psoriasis on my elbows and knees for years. Since I hate to take pills, I took a powedered-liquid vitamin. Within one year, all my psoriatic symptoms cleared up. My skin was smooth and healthy-looking. It was only by trial and error that I learned I was not receiving all the nutrients I thought I was getting. And again, I was eating well. Although this is anecdotal and to my knowledge there are no clinical studies to prove this, in my case this was highly significant. Even if we are not sick, we may unknowingly be in less than a state of perfect health.

FIGHTING RADIATION

I like to think of the body as a Porsche with a finely tuned engine requiring a high performance fuel to operate. When the fuel is of an inferior grade, the engine may spurt and sputter. When the engine has no fuel, it stops. The human body reacts in a similar fashion. We need food and nourishment in order to keep our engines going. However, if we do not give ourselves the proper nutrients, or insufficient nutrients, or perhaps even poor grade nutrients, our bodies will not function in a smooth and timely manner.

The problem with most of us is that we believe we are getting all we need from our diets. But is this true? Overcooking foods, for example, or microwaving them may alter the biochemical makeup of vitamins and enzymes. This, in a sense, is similar to using a low grade fuel. Freshness can also be fleeting. Frequently, fresh produce will lose much of its vitamin value because of storage, shipping, and handling. Asparagus, for example, loses up to two-thirds of its vitamin C just after two days of room temperature.

Although the vitamins and minerals found in natural whole foods will give us some protection against illness, I *do* believe that *supplementation enhances our health*. It is a little known fact, for example, that *certain vitamin and mineral supplements can significantly protect individuals against the increasing dangers of radiation and chemical pollutants.* As a clinical cardiologist, I have seen numerous articles on the beneficial effects of beta carotene, vitamins A, C, and E, as well as selenium. These nutrients are frequently referred to as antioxidants, which protect our bodies from the formation of free radicals sometimes associated with cancer.

Free radicals are unstable atoms or electrons that cause damage to our cells or can even kill them. They can break chemical bonds, thus impairing our immune systems and predisposing us to infections leading to various degenerative diseases. These unstable highly reactive molecules may be generated from within, resulting from metabolic reactions in the body or from outside sources such as air pollution, cigarette smoke and ionizing radiation. They frequently result from chemical pollutants and are side effects of radiation as well as to overexposure to the sun's rays. Since our environment is becoming more and more polluted, particularly by heavy metals such as cadmium, aluminum, lead, and mercury, and since the ozone layer is receding, our bodies are more prone to these harmful effects.

There is also considerable investigation into the impact of radon on the formation of free radicals, which seems to be a major factor in the development of lung cancer. Radon is found deep in the earth in rocks. Over time, the toxic effects of radon in our homes can infiltrate our bodies. For example, I have a patient with lung cancer who never smoked, but his home was contaminated with radon. As radon gas is radioactive, he is currently involved in a state-wide study to determine the degree of the relationship between radon and lung cancer. Environmental toxicities that can produce free radicals are all around us.

Unfortunately, free radicals can also be produced by the body itself, resulting from the oxidation of fat. When oxygen is utilized in the burning of fat (oxidation), the fat may turn rancid, thereby increasing free radical production.

In his provocative book, *Fighting Radiation with Foods, Herbs, and Vitamins,* Stephen R. Schechter discusses the damaging aspects of free radical formation. Like unguided missiles, free radicals attack cellular membranes without any rhyme or reason. In this process, accelerated cellular and eventually tissue break down occurs. In effect, he says antioxidants sacrifice themselves to free radicals by donating electrons and combining with these unstable atoms, thus causing the free radicals to stabilize. Such antioxidants as vitamins A, C, E, B-1, B-5, B-6, PABA, Coenzyme Q_{10}, and the minerals, zinc and selenium, are called free radical scavengers because of their neutralizing action in the body. Free radicals have been incriminated in such diseases as heart disease, cancer, emphysema, rheumatoid arthritis, cataracts, Parkinson disease, senility, and are considered by some to be the primary cause of aging.

Cataracts, for example, are the most common deterioration of aging. There are multiple clinical studies that indicate that prior treatment with antioxidizing agents, especially beta carotene may actually reduce cataract formation.

It is this free radical theory that so appeals to me as a doctor. Many of us, not only eat high-fat diets that can form free radicals, but we are also daily exposed to radiation. As a clinical cardiologist, I am frequently exposed to radiation. Performing cardiac catheterizations and inserting pacemakers, requires working with x-ray devices which produce radiation. The patient gets a small dose as well as the doctor. Since radiation accumulates over time, many small doses add up and can certainly be disruptive to the body. In my particular case, I stopped performing cardiac catheterizations because of hemorrhages found in my corneas that I believe were related to radiation.

HEALING POWER OF VITAMINS

After reading another article where vitamin A was noted to reduce the formation of cataracts, I seriously began to investigate vitamins and minerals as a way of self-healing. My investigation included computer searches and extensive reading, and upon its completion I *now believe in the benefits of vitamins, minerals, and foods that induce healing.* Although I continue to eat natural foods, I do take vitamin and mineral supplementation. Since we are all exposed to radiation or chemical pollutants in our environment that may be destructive to many vitamins as well as essential fatty acids, it is a good idea to try to protect ourselves with these added nutrients.

In addition, many of us consume fats, particularly fried foods, and most of us have eaten in fast-food restaurants where fats and oils are cooked at high temperatures. Remembering that the waste products of oxidized fats are toxic, it makes sense to supplement our diets with vitamins and minerals. Vitamins such as C, E, Beta Carotene, Q_{10}, and others offer an antioxidant defense against free radical invasion. It is this critical ingredient in winning the body's unrelenting biochemical war with our diets that is so essential in halting tissue deterioration.

But how much vitamin and mineral supplementation is enough? We need to be aware that the recommended daily allowance (RDA) was instituted *approximately 40-45 years ago* by the U.S. Food and Nutrition Board to determine the daily amount of vitamins and nutrients necessary to prevent illness directly due to vitamin deficiencies such as scurvy, beriberi, etc,. The RDA's, however, are considered to be only *minimal* doses that ward off such conditions, and these diseases are rare today. It has become apparent that larger doses of vitamins, but not megadoses, may provide more protection for the body. *The RDA may not be enough given today's radiation and chemically-polluted environment.* We need to consider a larger dose than the RDA recommendation to provide an optimal daily allowance that is health-enhancing.

Taking vitamins and minerals in their proper balance is important. For example, high doses of isolated B vitamins may cause depletion of other B vitamins, or too much of the mineral zinc may cause anemia. It was recently observed in the **Journal of the American Medical Association,** that large numbers of elderly patients who are given vitamins may be ingesting too much zinc. A careful history about zinc ingestion is necessary when evaluating elderly patients for anemia. We also need to be aware that some vitamin supplements, particularly vitamins A and D, can cause serious illnesses if taken in excess dosages. *The key here again is moderation.* Although a full discussion of vitamin and mineral supplementation is beyond the scope of this text, I would like to highlight some points that I feel are essential in our *Lose to Win* thinking.

VITAMINS

Vitamins are a group of organic compounds that regulate the metabolism of carbohydrates, proteins, and fats. Vitamins are considered micro-nutrients and act as a catalyst for chemical reactions in the body. Frequently, a vitamin will be described as a coenzyme because it works with enzymes in assisting biochemical functions. Since vitamins cannot be produced by the body, we rely on getting them through the diet and/or in vitamin and mineral supplements.

Some vitamins may be fat-soluble, such as A, D, E, and K, and do not need to be replenished on a daily basis, as the body can store them in the adipose tissue. The water-soluble vitamins, such as the B's and vitamin C, must be ingested on a daily basis, as they cannot be stored in the body.

VITAMIN A

Vitamin A is essential to prevent night blindness and the formation of cataracts. It is also important in the development of healthy bones, skin, hair, and mucous membranes. It enhances immunity and is important in epithelial tissue (skin and mucous membranes) maintenance and repair. As an antioxidant, vitamin A helps protect against the adverse effects of radiation and chemical pollutants. Although high doses of vitamin A can be utilized in infections and under conditions of physical or emotional stress, supplements of vitamin A should not be taken in high dosages for a long period of time, as it is a fat-soluble vitamin and can be stored in the body. There have been cases on record where megadose therapy resulted in hypervitaminosis A, causing liver damage, skin rash and brain dysfunction.

Pro-vitamin A, or beta carotene, is a precursor of vitamin A and is converted into vitamin A by the body. *Beta carotene is a yellowish compound contained in carrot juice, canteloupe, watercress, and other fruits and vegetables, especially those with yellow, orange, or dark green hues.* Unlike vitamin A, beta carotene has been shown to have little toxic side effects. Except for the tendency to turn the skin a slight yellow-orange color when used to an extreme, the only other caution should be in medically uncontrolled diabetic and hypothyroid individuals, as they have difficulty metabolizing beta carotene. Recently, beta carotene has become a fashionable vitamin. It has been supported by medical experts in a recent Harvard study as contributing to the prevention of cancer as well as coronary artery disease. Both vitamin A and beta carotene are extremely important in the immune mechanisms of the body and may help to fight the common cold and other flu-like illnesses. Beta Carotene also has been reported to protect the lung from increased ozone and smog in polluted city environments and is helpful in combating the toxic effects of automobile emissions.

The RDA for vitamin A or beta carotene is 3,000 IU's for children and 5,000 IU's for adults. We also get plenty of vitamin A in the diet. *Foods that contain considerable quantities of vitamin A include carrots, beets, cantaloupe, broccoli, Swiss chard, dandelion greens, garlic, kale, parsley, red peppers, sweet potatoes, spinach, yellow squash, turnip greens, and watercress.* For an animal source of vitamin A, I recommend *fish liver oils, particularly cod liver oil, as I do not recommend eating calves liver or other organ meats.* Although I'm sure vitamin supplements would be preferable, one tablespoon of cod liver oil contains 11,000 units of pre-formed vitamin A. Similarly, three and one-half ounces of carrots offer approximately 11,500 units of vitamin A. It is also important to note that antibiotics, cholesterol-lowering agents, some laxatives, various antacids, and excessive quantities of alcohol or caffeine may interfere with vitamin A absorption.

Vitamin B complex with vitamin B-1 (thiamin)

My first exposure to a patient with vitamin B-1 deficiency occurred during my internship. A man in his mid-fifties presented to the Albany Medical Center Hospital with congestive heart failure. He reminded me of "Popeye." His arms and legs were very swollen and he was suffering from chronic heart failure. This man was an alcoholic. Although he responded to the usual treatment for heart failure at the time, i.e. diuretics and Digoxin (a heart-strengthening medicine), he did not appear to improve significantly until he received vitamin B-1. Thiamin enhances the circulation and is needed for the normal functioning of the heart muscle and smooth muscle of the gastrointestinal tract. It is also an important constituent for the central nervous system. *Excellent sources of vitamin B-1 include brown rice, whole grains, green vegetables, peas, wheat germ, soybeans, dried beans, green vegetables, brussels sprouts, oatmeal, prunes, raisins, and sunflower seeds, to mention a few.*

Vitamin B-2 (riboflavin)

Riboflavin is necessary for antibody production, cell respiration, and metabolism of fats, carbohydrates, and proteins. Signs of riboflavin deficiency include cracks and sores at the corner of the mouth. It also has been suggested by researchers that riboflavin may alleviate allergic conjunctivitis, a common problem for hay fever sufferers. It is also beneficial for the skin, nails, and hair. It may be helpful in controlling dandruff. *Sources of riboflavin include leafy green vegetables, whole grains, spinach, poultry, fish, meat, asparagus, broccoli, brussels sprouts, currants, and sea vegetables.* It is also important to know that oral contraceptives may increase the need for riboflavin, and this is one particular vitamin that is easily destroyed by overcooking and use of alcohol.

VITAMIN B-3 (NIACIN)

Niacin is an important vitamin for circulation, energy production, and functioning of the nervous system. In large doses, it is helpful in lowering cholesterol. My first personal experience with niacin was rather unusual. I took niacin in the powdered form, only to realize that instead of taking the instruction of teaspoons, I took tablespoons. I immediately developed a "niacin flush" accompanied by the tingling of the skin associated with a hot flash. I really thought I was having an allergic reaction. I immediately went back to one of my textbooks on niacin and found that this is a sensation which, to my surprise, was welcomed by many people who experience it. Large amounts of niacin, however, can be injurious, particularly to the liver. Deficiencies in niacin may cause abnormalities in the central nervous system *Excellent sources of niacin include meat products, broccoli, grains, dried beans, potatoes, tomatoes, and nuts.*

VITAMIN B-5 (PANTOTHENIC ACID)

Pantothenic acid, also referred to as vitamin B-5, is known as the "anti-stress vitamin" because of its crucial role in energy metabolism. Under situations of severe emotional and physical stress, it is not uncommon for some individuals to need an additional 500 mg of pantothenic acid per day. Although the human requirement for pantothenic acid is not known, 10 mg is considered sufficient. However, more of the vitamin is required after injury, stress, or during antibiotic therapy. Although symptoms of pantothenic acid deficiency are rare, considerable amounts of the vitamin are lost in the processing, canning, and cooking of foods, especially in acidic or alkaline solutions.

The brain contains the highest concentration of pantothenic acid in the body, therefore, a deficiency of pantothenic acid, like all the B vitamins, would include symptoms such as easy fatiguability, depression, and insomnia. The alcoholic is one individual who may be particularly prone to B vitamin deficiency, especially if foods are not consumed. *Excellent sources of pantothenic acid would include whole grains, meat, cabbage, cauliflower, beans, eggs, saltwater fish, and poultry.*

VITAMIN B-6 (PYRIDOXINE)

Vitamin B-6 is an important vitamin in the regulation and formation of blood cells. It is required for the synthesis of nucleic acids. Some investigators reported that vitamin B-6 helped some individuals recall dreams. It also has been used to calm the effects of premenstrual syndrome and is helpful in the treatment of allergies and asthma. In weight loss, B6 has been reported to be a useful nutrient. Oral contraceptives may increase the need for vitamin B-6. The urologist may prescribe vitamin B-6, as it is useful in preventing calcium oxalate gravel in the urinary tract. In short, vitamin B-6 is an important coenzyme in the metabolism of amino acids that can affect our mental and physical health. Most foods contain small amounts of vitamin B-6. *The best sources, however, include green vegetables, brewers' yeast, carrots, fish, meat, peas, sunflower seeds, avocados, and green peppers.*

VITAMIN B-12 (CYANOCOBALAMIN)

Vitamin B-12 is necessary in the formation of blood cells and actually prevents anemia. It is also necessary in the maintenance of a healthy nervous system. A prolonged absence of vitamin B-12 may cause pernicious anemia. This is a type of anemia that may cause weakness and lethargy and damage to the nervous system. I remember one of my elderly patients who had an absorption problem with vitamin B-12. When he presented in my office with angina, he almost underwent coronary artery bypass surgery because of his severe coronary disease. We discovered, however, that his angina possibly could have been provoked by a low blood count resulting from a vitamin B-12 deficiency. After he received vitamin B-12 injections, he felt considerably better with less symptoms of angina. He now visits his family physician on a monthly basis to obtain B-12 shots which completely corrected the problem. He has been with this particular treatment for approximately three years and, at the age of 77, has a good quality of life. *Sources of vitamin B-12 include all animal foods, cheese, eggs, milk, tofu, and sea vegetables. Since B-12 is not found in most vegetables, vegetarians need to be cautious and supplement B-12 in their diet.*

OTHER B VITAMINS

Other B complex vitamins include biotin, choline, folic acid, inositol, and para-aminobenzoic acid (PABA). These vitamins are found in many of the foods mentioned in vitamins B-12 with the exception of PABA, which is found in molasses, liver, and kidney, as well as whole grains. Para-aminobenzoic acid is an antioxidant which may protect against sunburn and various skin cancers. Since most preparations of B vitamins include a multi-B complex, and are water-soluble, it is only necessary to take these in small doses on a daily basis, as the excess amount is excreted. Generally, there are no known toxicities if the B vitamins are taken in small amounts. In large amounts, however, one has to utilize caution, particularly with vitamin B-3, which can be injurious to the liver. There are no known side effects for vitamin B-5, pantothenic acid. It is also important to note that alcohol and caffeine, as well as birth control pills and estrogen replacements, can have a negative impact on B vitamins. Caffeine and alcohol, for example, may affect the elimination of B vitamins and oral contraceptives or estrogens may result in a functional deficiency of the B vitamins. This is related to complex hormonal pathways in which relative B-6 and B-12 deficiencies may occur. Thus, in patients on estrogen, it is reasonable to meet the body's increased need for B-2, B-6, and B-12 with nutritional supplements.

VITAMIN C

Vitamin C has been the subject of considerable controversy over the last few years, particularly when Linus Pauling first publicized it as the "cure for the common cold." Numerous research studies have indicated that vitamin C improves the immune system. In the animal model, for example, vitamin C has been known to protect against lethal doses of radiation. Perhaps the most famous and noteworthy effects of vitamin C are on preventing the disease scurvy. Scurvy is an illness in which subcutaneous bleeding occurs along with a loss of appetite, tender joints, and a low grade anemia accompanied by slow wound healing. Centuries ago, sailing ships used to carry limes in order to prevent scurvy. Vitamin C is a powerful antioxidant that is necessary for tissue growth and repair, particularly in the gums.

Vitamin C also plays a crucial role in the absorption of iron, which is necessary for the formation of red blood cells, thereby preventing anemia. Doctors frequently administer vitamin C in combination with iron to increase the iron assimilation in the body. Vitamin C creates a favorable acidic pH in the stomach so that iron-bound compounds can be absorbed. Vitamin C is also an essential constituent in the metabolism of amino acids, particularly tyrosine and phenylalanine.

During psychological and emotional stress, vitamin C may become depleted from the adrenal glands. Dietary supplementation with foods rich in vitamin C or vitamin supplements may help prevent the body's negative reaction to prolonged stress. Some clinical studies have also demonstrated a reduction in serum cholesterol with vitamin C supplementation. Since the body cannot manufacture its own vitamin C, it must be obtained through the diet or in nutritional supplements. E–sterified and timed release preparations may be more bio available and thus more effective at the tissue level. Since most vitamin C is water-soluble and can be expelled in the urine, it needs to be taken on a daily basis.

Common sources of vitamin C include green leafy vegetables, bell peppers, broccoli, squash, cabbage, strawberries, lemons, kale, grapefruit, oranges, currants, parsley, onions, green peas, radishes, rosehips, spinach, Swiss chard, tomatoes, turnip greens, and brussels sprouts.

Once again, it is important for us to remember that oral contraceptives and corticosteroids may reduce the levels of vitamin C in the body. Alcohol is also an antagonist to vitamin C. Although symptoms of a toxicity are rare with high intakes of vitamin C, kidney stones could occur if vitamin C is taken in large doses and not accompanied by adequate hydration. In doses greater than 5,000 mg a day, some side effects may occur. Excess urination, diarrhea, or skin rashes may be experienced as some tolerable side effects.

VITAMIN D

Vitamin D is the bone vitamin. A deficiency of vitamin D may impair the growth and development of bone structures. This is commonly seen in the pathologic entity called rickets in children and osteomalacia in adults. In addition to bone, the maintenance of healthy teeth is enhanced by vitamin D. *The principle source of vitamin D comes from the sun's ultraviolet rays.* A deficiency of vitamin D could result from lack of exposure to the sun, especially if the natural vitamin is not taken in the diet. Nursing home inhabitants, for example, who do not wish to go out into the sun are susceptible to vitamin D deficiency.

This is an important consideration since vitamin D is not self-activated and requires conversion by the liver, in either its natural or supplement form. Routine sunshine, perhaps as little as one-half hour per day, is all that is necessary to activate the vitamin D metabolism in the body. It is also important to note that in the elderly, vitamin D can help in the overall treatment of osteoporosis, an illness resulting from gradual loss of bone, predominantly in the spine and hips, that affects approximately 25 percent of women over the age of 50. When treating osteoporosis, it is important to know the overall health of the patient. Many of these individuals may have kidney and liver disease or are frequently diabetic. Thus, vitamin and mineral supplementation is critical in this population.

As vitamin D is a fat-soluble vitamin and, therefore, may be stored in the body, it may be toxic if taken in megadoses. This can be particularly serious in children or in individuals with kidney disease. Some drugs, such as steroid hormones, interfere with the action of vitamin D in the intestines while others, such as cholesterol-lowering drugs, may also interfere with the absorption of vitamin D. The dietary sources of vitamin D include *fish oils and saltwater fish, especially fatty fish like halibut, salmon, mackerel, and bluefish. It is also found in abundance in eggs, liver, milk, sweet potatoes, and sunflower seeds.*

VITAMIN E

For the cardiologist, vitamin E is gaining more and more popularity. An article concerning vitamin E and its inverse relationship to angina was recently published in the prestigious medical journal *Lancet.* Vitamin C and beta carotene were also cited as being beneficial in treating angina. Although the mechanism for vitamin E and its protective effects on the heart are not well established, recent research indicates that vitamin E is an important antioxidant that may help protect unsaturated fatty acids from breaking down and causing the formation of free radicals. Vitamin E may help lower the deleterious influence of LDL on cellular membranes. In addition, it has been reported to aid

111

against the long-term effects of aging and may be used as an adjunct in cancer treatments.

The favorable effects of vitamin E on the immune system were demonstrated in an animal study using lethal doses of radiation. In one particular study, two groups of mice were radiated. One was given vitamin E and the other not. The mice who were radiated but not given vitamin E succumbed to the radiation. The experimental group, however, had an increase in survival, thereby showing the protective effects of vitamin E against radiation and on the overall immune response. Vitamin E has been shown to be effective against many common pollutants in the environment such as nitroamines (carcinogens found in many processed meats), chlorine, mercury, and carbon monoxide. In the medical literature, reporting on vitamin E is becoming more and more common. The once thought of "sex vitamin" is now standing on its own as an effective healing agent, not only for its merits in cancer and cardiovascular disease, but also in its effectiveness as an antipollutant vitamin. With beta carotene and Vitamin C in combination, Vitamin E is extremely helpful in neutralizing the deleterious effects of industrial pollutants and toxic heavy metals.

Vitamin E has also been reported to be effective in thinning the blood, eliminating leg cramps, and aiding in the prevention of cataracts, as well as decreasing the breast tenderness and swelling experienced in the PMS syndrome. The best sources of vitamin E include *vegetable oils such as wheat germ oil and peanut oil. Green leafy vegetables, nuts, seeds, dry beans, brown rice, and whole wheat are other good sources of vitamin E.* As a supplement, approximately 400 units of vitamin E per day is suggested to enhance the body's health and immunity. Although not all the mechanisms of vitamin E are clear, medical research has revealed yet another secret of the role of vitamin E in health. It has recently been discovered that vitamin E's role may be important in increasing the production of coenzyme Q_{10}.

COENZYME Q_{10}

*One of the most exciting and intriguing insights that I learned in researching this book was the personal discovery and health benefits of Q_{10}. Actually, I first learned about Q_{10} several years ago in an article that appeared in the **Annals of Thoracic Surgery** in February of 1982.*

In this particular study, a control group and an experimental group were designed to investigate the impact of Q_{10} on cardiovascular heart function in patients placed on the heart-lung machine during open heart surgery. The article concluded that patients given Q_{10} prior to open heart surgery actually had an improvement in their heart functions. It also reported that the preoperative administration of this vitamin-like substance could favorably increase one's tolerance to the low oxygen state that occurs during open heart surgery. Thus, Q_{10} increased cardiac output and overall heart efficiency.

Although this study was highly provocative, my openness to such vitamin and mineral therapy at that time, to say the least, was nonexistent. As a well-trained traditional cardiologist, I saw no need for such nutritional supplementation, particularly since drugs such as Digitalis, diuretics, and other myocardial stimulants were considered highly useful. It took several years of experience, growth, and humility to teach me that vitamins and other natural remedies can be a useful adjunct to traditional medical therapies.

Congestive heart failure is a term that cardiologists refer to as a weakening of the heart muscle. When the heart muscle becomes so weak that it cannot pump the blood effectively to the organs of the body, patients may develop swelling of the ankles, lack of appetite, fatigue, and shortness of breath on activity. Sometimes the pumping ability of the heart is so impaired that the blood, instead of being pumped out of the heart, backs up into the lungs. At this time patients will complain of shortness of breath during activities and sometimes at rest, especially while lying down. Congestive heart failure is a failing heart or an energy-starved heart. For all practical purposes, the tiny myocardial cells are so exhausted that they cannot sustain sufficient intrinsic cellular energy, thus they cannot contract and effectively create a pumping mechanism for the blood to be circulated around the body. Congestive heart failure is indeed the most frustrating and challenging dilemma of my profession.

Over the last 20 years I have seen hundreds of patients with congestive heart failure. For some, the diagnosis is obvious; that is, if a large heart attack destroys a considerable quantity of heart muscle, the contracting action of the heart is so impaired that the remaining viable myocardial cells eventually become exhausted and worn out in sustaining the circulatory pumping action of the heart.

Similarly, a long-standing history of high blood pressure can also impair such myocardial function. Valvular disease, frequently induced by childhood rheumatic fever, as well as viral illnesses and toxins such as chronic alcohol abuse, can likewise impair the functioning of the heart muscle. As a clinical cardiologist, I can also attest to numerous cases of unexplained heart failure. These are individuals who have "cardiomyopathy" of an unknown nature; that is, in these individuals, there was no known cause of heart muscle weakening. There was no history of diabetes, heart attack, high blood pressure, alcohol abuse, rheumatic fever, or severe viral illnesses. Some patients just develop weakening of the heart from no apparent cause. Some of the cardiomyopathies have also been found to be due to a nutritional origin. Vitamin deficiencies such as beriberi, thiamine deficiency, and the rare postpartum cardiomyopathy of pregnancy may be related to nutritional deficiencies that have been known to cause congestive heart failure.

Although some patients with cardiomyopathy improve, the majority of these individuals deteriorate. For the cardiologist, the treatment of heart failure is similar to the oncologist treating a life threatening cancer. Although we can find drugs to help control symptoms, there is really no known cure for cardiomyopathy. Like some form of incurable cancer, there is frequently a deterioration that ultimately ends in death. One of the most heartbreaking weeks of my practice occurred approximately one year prior to writing this book. During that one week period, I lost five male patients from congestive heart failure. Many of these patients were my clients and also my "friends" for several years.

NEW HOPE

My rediscovery of Q_{10} in the preparation of this manuscript has now given me an exciting charge of optimism that may offer an improvement in quality of life and hope in the treatment of these patients! It is true that in February of 1982, a very favorable article was reported in a major cardiology journal. But most of my colleagues and I probably did not really appreciate the true meaning of this article. Even when I was preparing for this manuscript, I really did not place too much emphasis on Q_{10}.

Then, one of my colleagues in endocrinology, Dr. Lester Kritzer, questioned me about the healing properties of the coenzyme. He then gave me a book entitled *The Miracle Nutrient Coenzyme Q_{10}* by Emile G. Bliznakof, M.D. and Gerald L. Hunt. After reading the exciting contents of the book, and particularly after looking at the bibliography, I began to inquire about Q_{10}. I went to the library and requested major articles that were listed in the cardiology literature. As I read some of these articles, I became excited and also intrigued.

Surprisingly, another timely and fortuitous event happened. One of the most reknowned cardiologists in the world was speaking at our hospital as I was reviewing the literature on Q_{10}. As the Director of Medical Education, I had invited Dr. William Frishman, a Professor of Medicine at Albert Einstein College of Medicine, to address our medical staff on high blood pressure in the geriatric population. As we were chatting a few minutes prior to his discussion, he inquired about what I was doing with my life. He knew of my training as a psychotherapist with a special interest in the emotional aspects of heart disease. I shared with him my development of this book on nutritional and emotional healing. I then directed him to my inquiries about coenzyme Q_{10}. His energy changed and his eyes lit up. Not only did he know about Q_{10}, but he had published a major article in the respected journal **Medical Clinics of North America** on cardiovascular pharmacology in January 1988.

I almost fell off my chair! He also proceeded to tell me that Q_{10}, in his clinical studies, was considered therapeutic not only in congestive heart failure, but cardiac arrhythmia, and high blood pressure as well! My interest was now overwhelming. I became so excited about this fortuitous discovery that I was determined to learn all I could about this nutrient. I then proceeded to request our Pharmacy Department to place it on formulary and furthermore to disseminate information to the medical staff about its use.

Why Haven't You Heard About Q_{10}?

But why has the discovery of Q_{10} not made more of an impact on physicians? The answer can probably be traced to two reasons. First of all, Q_{10} was not identified until 1940. It was not until the mid 1960's that it was first demonstrated to be of use in the treatment of cardiovascular disease. Thus, it is a very recent discovery in the medical world. Clinicians, in general, are not very open to the healing properties of natural vitamins, herbs, and coenzymes. Admittedly, I, too, was not very interested in Q_{10} after my first exposure to it 10 years ago. But after becoming a bioenergetic analyst over the last 12 years and studying the impact energy has on the organism, I came to realize the profound importance of the energetic principle, especially at the cellular level. This appreciation left me with an unquenchable thirst for the subsequent investigation of Q_{10}.

So enough of all this. *What is Q_{10}?* Q-enzyme ten is a vitamin-like substance that is similar in structure to vitamin K. Like vitamin E, it is a powerful antioxidant. In humans, Q_{10} is found in high concentrations in various organs, particularly the heart which has its highest concentration. In cells, the highest concentration of Q_{10} is found primarily in the mitochondria or so-called powerhouses that supply energy to the cell.

The function of Q_{10} is to stabilize cell membranes and act as an antioxidant and free radical scavenger in preventing the depletion of products necessary for the production of adenosine triphosphate (ATP). ATP is needed in almost every energy transaction in the body. Thus, Q_{10} is needed to enhance the production of cellular energy by stimulating the formation of ATP at the mitochondrial level. Q_{10} is critical for the production of energy and healthy functioning of the cell.

Since Q_{10} is necessary for the optimal functioning of the cell, can a deficiency of Q_{10} impair such energy production? The answer to that question is *yes*. An intriguing speculation can therefore be raised. Can cardiovascular malfunction such as congestive heart failure be caused by a deficiency of Q_{10}? The answer to that question is also *yes*.

The father of Q_{10} research, Dr. Carl Folklers, demonstrated that patients with cardiovascular disease are deficient in Q_{10}. He found that levels of Q_{10} in cardiac patients are lower than in age-matched controls. Moreover, Folklers has also determined through autopsy and biopsy studies on both diseased and healthy human hearts that once internal levels of Q_{10} drop below 25 percent of normal, disease may develop. If levels drop below 75 percent, serious pathology and even death may occur. Although more research needs to be done, Folkler predicts that Q_{10} therapy will be an accepted international treatment for congestive heart failure.

For instance, Japanese and more recently USA studies have shown the favorable impact of supplementing Q_{10} to individuals with congestive heart failure. By increasing the level of intrinsic cellular energy, Q_{10} has a direct and beneficial effect on the energy-depleted muscle cells of the failing heart. Since Q_{10} protects critical cellular components from low oxygen states, the administration of Q_{10} thereby enhances the energy production in a cell and an organ that is literally starving for energy. Since it has been demonstrated that Q_{10} declines with advancing age, perhaps idiopathic cardiomyopathy may be related to a deficiency of cellular and mitochondrial Q_{10}.

For some unexplained reason the body's ability to extract Q_{10} from natural food sources declines with the aging of the organs, the liver being the most significant. Supplemental Q_{10} may be a significant healing remedy in selected populations especially the elderly. In experimental animal studies, administered Q_{10} protected heart cells from the damaging effects of oxygen deficiency. There are also multiple clinical studies to show that Q_{10} protects individuals from the chest pain or discomfort that doctors frequently refer to as angina pectoris. Exercise studies, for example, in patients with angina pectoris, have shown longer duration of exercise time in patients treated with coenzyme Q_{10}.

The protective effects for angina probably come from Q_{10}'s increased resynthesis of ATP, thereby increasing energy production and oxygen delivery. The utility of coenzyme Q_{10} in the treatment of angina pectoris and congestive heart failure has been demonstrated in multiple double blind and placebo controlled studies. The cardiovascular literature has also demonstrated a reduction in blood pressure as well. Apparently, some hypertensive patients may be deficient in coenzyme Q_{10}. In one placebo controlled double blind study, patients given Q_{10} demonstrated a reduction in both systolic and diastolic blood pressures over matched controls.

OTHER BENEFITS

We have spoken about the myocardial protective effects of coenzyme Q_{10} during open heart surgery. In addition, coenzyme Q_{10} has also been found to be an anti-arrhythmic agent. This has been demonstrated in both animal and human studies. Q_{10} has also been used in treating other disorders. For example, some forms of muscular dystrophy have been known to respond to Q_{10} therapy. In addition, Q_{10} has been used in the treatment of periodontal disease and has recently been used in bolstering the effects of the immune system and thus has been utilized in the treatment of immunodeficiency diseases. The use of Q_{10} in the AIDS syndrome will need further investigation.

Weight reduction is yet another useful attribute of Q_{10}. In my counseling of patients about weight reduction, it became apparent that some patients actually did adhere to a diet, but could not lose weight. Perhaps these patients did not burn calories, possibly as a result of a lower metabolism. In one European study, obese patients were found to be deficient in Q_{10}. As in congestive heart failure, this raises more intriguing speculation. Could Q_{10} be a helpful adjunct in diet therapy? Although this may appear to be speculative, the use of Q_{10} in selective individuals with presumed low metabolism may appear to be quite useful. An anecdotal case comes to mind. Mary, a woman in her fifties, came to our weight reducing program out of frustration because she had tried several programs before. She had a tremendous inability to lose weight. Although her resistance was apparent both on psychological and physical levels, her conscious drive continued her persistent struggle for weight loss. Unexpectedly, after two weeks on our high fiber, low fat program, Mary lost no weight. At that point I sensed her tremendous despair. She was really trying. After carefully going over her *Lose to Win* program, it was apparent that she was "staying on the diet". At this point, I suggested some dietary supplements that would enhance her metabolism. I placed her on a formula of Q_{10}, Vitamin B6, zinc, glucose tolerance factor, and a multi-vitamin and mineral complex. She was told to take these supplements after every meal. She persisted in her high fiber, low fat regimen and, to her surprise, had lost five pounds in the following week. According to the group leader who counseled Mary, this was the first time in several years that she lost the weight. Perhaps, as others, she may have had a low metabolism and in addition, perhaps a subtle deficiency in selected vitamin and mineral nutrients. At the end of this chapter, various formulas for vitamin and mineral supplementation will be addressed.

Clinical research has also revealed the use of coenzyme Q_{10} has multiple beneficial effects in brain disorders, aging, and in situations of allergy. For example, Q_{10} has the ability to counteract histamine and may have considerable utility in the treatment of asthma.

The usual dose of Q_{10} may range from 10-30 mg three times a day to up to 100-150 mg in pharmacological doses for the treatment of congestive heart failure, angina, and hypertension. In clinical studies where

150 mg has been used, no significant side effects have occurred. In a large study of over 5000 patients taking a dose of 30 mg, abdominal discomfort was reported in 20 patients and loss of appetite in 12. Since Q_{10} is neither a protein nor a foreign substance, little serious side effects can be anticipated.

The best sources of Q_{10} are usually found in red meat such as beef and pork. Other good sources of Q_{10} would include mackerel, salmon, sardines, eggs, wheat germ, spinach, and broccoli. Since the highest concentrations of Q_{10} are found in red meats, particularly organ meats, this usually may create an undesirable deficiency, particularly for the cardiac patient who is discouraged from eating red meats, organs (liver), and eggs. Therefore, *supplements are probably necessary,* especially in the elderly and those on vegetarian-type diets.

I personally take between 30 and 60 milligrams of coenzyme Q_{10} per day. I take the vitamin for several reasons. First of all, as a physician, I encounter many individuals with flu-like illnesses. As a cardiologist, I am frequently faced with stressful events such as radiation and life threatening situations. I take Q_{10} to bolster my immunity and, in addition, to prevent the oxidation of harmful LDL in my blood vessels. I also do not eat many foods that contain Q_{10} with the exception of broccoli and salmon. My own personal experience with Q_{10} has been extremely favorable, to say the least. My allergies have improved, particularly allergic conjunctivitis. My experience with my patients has also been extremely rewarding. To this date, I have well over 200 patients on Q_{10} therapy. I also have had several patients, for example, with cardiac arrhythmias who were reluctant to take standard antiarrhythmic drugs because of persistent side effects. One patient who suffered from a "panic disorder" was continuously plagued by cardiac irregularities. It was not uncommon for him to go to the emergency room on several occasions because of an irregular heart beat. Since Q_{10} therapy, his admissions to the emergency room have ceased. For another patient with congestive heart failure, the addition of Q_{10} had a considerable impact on his quality of life. This poor individual was functioning at a daily life routine of going from bed to a chair. With the use of Q_{10}, he was able to walk and function with much less shortness of breath. His quality of life improved tremendously with the addition of Q_{10} to his usual medical therapies. Many others have also responded as favorably.

Thus, in the cardiovascular patient the use of Q_{10} may serve as a valuable adjunct in therapy, with minimal risk of side effects. In addition to the treatment of heart disease, Q_{10} may have beneficial effects in cancer and obesity, as well as the immunodeficiency diseases. It is also interesting to note that Q_{10} has been officially approved by the ministry of health in Japan and is on formulary in all Japanese hospitals. Since there is overwhelming medical evidence supporting the the use of Q_{10} and neglible if any risk, it is my recommendation that this nutrient be utilized in treating many of the common degenerative, nutritional, and infectious diseases of the 20th century.

So, where can I get Q_{10}? And how much does it cost? In my own experience of soliciting many health food stores, I was able to find Q_{10} in perhaps two-thirds of the stores I visited. In grocery stores where vitamins are sold, I have yet to find one grocery store or chain that included Q_{10} in their product line. Manufacturers will sell Q_{10} in its pure form or use it in combination with a multi-vitamin and mineral combination. When Q_{10} is purchased, make sure that it is a yellow color, especially since Q_{10} in its pure form is yellow. The price of Q_{10} varies from one health food store to another. Although there have been several hundred articles in the medical literature on Q_{10}, one is to keep in mind that the FDA has not studied Q_{10} and, therefore, it is not considered a drug. If the FDA investigates Q_{10}, it could possibly be taken off the market and regulated under the auspices of the FDA. If such is the case, the cost of this nutrient could go considerably higher, particularly if a doctor's prescription is necessary and if the "vitamin" is only sold at pharmacies. It is my hope that this will not happen since this could place an unnecessary economic burden on those wishing to take this vitamin on a daily basis.

MINERALS

Like vitamins, minerals perform many functions in the body that are essential to our health, particularly at the cellular level. They are important components of bone and blood, and help to maintain healthy nerve and organ function. Minerals are inorganic substances that come from rock formations deep in the earth. After the breakdown of rocks by erosion, minerals are then passed from the rocks to the soil and then to plants and the rest of the food chain. *If you eat whole foods and simply wash the vegetable skins as opposed to peeling them, the absorption of vitamins and minerals will be greater.*

It is important to note that once minerals are absorbed, they may be in competition with each other. Excessive zinc can deplete the body of copper, for example, and excessive calcium can affect magnesium and manganese absorption. We also need to consider that individuals on high-fiber diets containing phytate, a binding agent, may risk mineral deficiency when the mineral intake is low or borderline low. High fiber may decrease transit time in the intestines resulting in a decrease in mineral absorption. Thus, high fiber diets and/or vegetarian diets may require additional mineral supplementation. When taking mineral supplements, it is important to take a multisupplement rather than individual high dosage, unless recommended by your physician.

A full discussion of minerals is beyond the scope of this book. As with vitamins, I will try to emphasize the overall importance of several of the major minerals and their usefulness in some of the common medical syndromes that doctors frequently see, such as osteoporosis and chronic fatigue syndrome.

TABLE 12

RECOMMENDED DAILY DIETARY ALLOWANCES FOR CALCIUM

AGE OR CONDITION	CALCIUM
1-10 years	800 mg
11-24 years	1,200 mg
25-50 years	800 mg
51 years and older	800 mg
Pregnancy	1,200 mg
Lactating (first year)	1,200 mg

1989 Food and Nutrition Board, National Academy of Science/National Research Council

CALCIUM

Calcium is an important mineral and is necessary for good bone and teeth development. It is also a major mineral in cardiac electrical conduction and the transmission of impulses through the nerves. It is needed for the contraction of muscles and is essential in blood clotting. Calcium deficiencies may cause muscle cramps, cardiac arrhythmia, brittle nails, tooth decay, and numbness in the arms and legs. The most critical period for adequate calcium intake is in childhood when the skeleton is developing. The recommended daily requirement for children is 800 to 1,200 mg per day (**Table 12**). It is also crucial for women to take the RDA minimum since they are at risk of developing osteoporosis, particularly in the postmenopausal state.

Calcium taken in the diet slows aging bone loss, and recent evidence indicates that providing calcium supplements to postmenopausal women does allow for slower bone loss whether or not they are combined with hormone replacement. Whatever age, women and men should aim to meet recommended dietary allowance for calcium. The absorption of calcium is variable. Usually only 20-30 percent of the calcium taken in in our diet is absorbed into the blood. Caffeine may limit its absorption, as may refined foods or foods grown in calcium-deficient soil.

The best sources of calcium include dairy products, seafood, green leafy vegetables except lettuce, asparagus, broccoli, cabbage, molasses, and sea vegetables (**Table 13**). *Sea vegetables are among the richest sources of calcium and magnesium in the world.* One ounce of wakame seaweed, for example, has approximately the same amount of calcium as eight ounces of milk. *Other wonderful sources of calcium include figs, dates, parsley, prunes and sesame seeds.* Utilizing sesame seeds as a accent in our foods is extremely healthful. These can be used when marinating fish or chicken, as well as in salads or on a bowl of rice. One cup of sesame seeds has as much calcium as three cups of milk.

Cheeses provide tremendous sources of calcium, but they are also a major source of fat. Cream cheese, for example, provides significant quantities of calcium but also has approximately 11 grams of fat per one ounce serving. Similarly, ice cream provides abundant calcium, but also considerable fat. Some gourmet ice creams, for example, may contain as much as 34 grams of fat per serving with 150 mg of calcium. *Low-fat frozen yogurts,* on the other hand, contain very little fat and the same amount of calcium. *Skim milk and very low-fat milk products are excellent sources of calcium that do not contain the excessive fat.* Here again, awareness is necessary. All milk, regardless of whether we are discussing whole milk, two percent, one percent, or even skim milk for that matter, provides about 300 mg of calcium per cup.

When taking calcium supplements, it is important to remember to take them throughout the day and before bedtime. Too much calcium, however, can be harmful. Prolonged high intake of calcium and vitamin D has been shown to cause hypercalcemia, which can affect one's blood pressure as well as kidney function. It is also important to note that excessive calcium may impair the absorption of zinc and manganese. Calcium supplements should be utilized with caution in anyone with kidney disease or advanced diabetes.

TABLE 13

FOODS HIGH IN CALCIUM

Cereals	Vegetables
Oatmeal (Quaker Instant)	Asparagus
Cheese	Broccoli
Feta	Cabbage
**Ricotta, Part skin	**Daikon
Fruits	Turtle beans
**Figs	Collards
Dates	**Kale
Prunes	Kelp
Milk/Yogurt	Parsley
**Skim milk	Wakame
**Lo-fat yogurt	**Tofu
**Skim yogurt	White beans
One percent milk	**Nuts and Seeds**
	Sesame seeds
	Soybean nuts

(** Foods Highest in Calcium)

ZINC

Zinc, an essential trace mineral, has many functions. The most important is probably on the prostate gland and growth of the reproductive organs. It is also important to the immune system, particularly in the healing of wounds. Zinc is necessary for the absorption and maintenance of vitamin E as well as the B-complex vitamins. Zinc is also an important mineral in helping the body eliminate toxic heavy metals such as aluminum, lead, and excess copper. It is now noted to be important in wound healing particularly in diabetics. *It is found in abundance in fish, meats, poultry, and whole grains.* Alcohol consumption, diuretics, excess calcium, or diarrhea may lower zinc levels.

Recently it has been shown that a deficiency in zinc may be related to excess fat storage, thus increasing weight gain. Zinc is therefore an important mineral to consider in weight reduction in its relation to glucose metabolism. In zinc deficiency states, sugars may be only partially metabolized leading to an increase availability for fat production and storage. In a pediatric study of overweight children having low levels of zinc, weight loss was retarded until zinc was supplemented in the diet. *Therefore, zinc may be important to investigate in individuals who are resistant to weight loss despite a thorough medical examination and modification of lifestyle and nutritional habits.*

MAGNESIUM

The recognition of magnesium is increasing, especially in the cardiovascular literature. Magnesium deficiency can result in a host of cardiological disorders including life threatening arrhythmias, heart muscle disease, and potentially fatal heart attack (**Table 14**). *As a cardiologist, I cannot overemphasize the importance of magnesium.* Cardiologists are well aware that magnesium deficiency is a leading cause of cardiac arrythmia in the presence of potassium depletion that fails to respond to usual therapies. It is well known, for example, that low magnesium states will significantly exacerbate the pro-arrhythmic effect of low serum potassium, especially in patients taking an excess of digitalis preparations (digoxin, lanoxin). Usually potassium and magnesium depletion are commonly present and the treatment is administering both agents.

Recently, the medical literature has also cited low red blood cell magnesium levels as a potential cause of the chronic fatigue syndrome.

Chronic fatigue syndrome is characterized by the presence of fatigue for more than six months, impairment of memory and concentration, and a variety of symptoms such as muscle aches, muscle tenderness, joint pain, headaches, and depression. Although the cause is generally unknown, a generalized immune deficiency seems to be a major factor. Viral illnesses, for example, have also been known to cause chronic fatigue. Usually the treatment of such a condition includes rest, alleviation of stress, and vitamin and nutritional therapy.

TABLE 14

POTENTIAL CARDIOVASCULAR CONSEQUENCES OF MAGNESIUM DEFICIENCY

- Cardiac arrhythmias (Abnormal rhythm)
- Coronary atherosclerosis
- Cardiomyopathy (Failure of the heart muscle)
- Coronary vasospasm (Chest pain)
- Heart attack
- Sudden death

In one particular study, some chronic fatigue syndrome patients were treated with magnesium and another group was given placebos. The magnesium treated patients reported heightened energy levels when compared with controls. Red cell magnesium levels were normalized in all the treated patients compared with only one control. Thus, magnesium has a potential role in the treatment of chronic fatigue syndrome. In another recent magnesium study, supplementation was proven to be an effective treatment of the premenstrual syndrome. In this double-blind placebo controlled study, both pain and mood change were positively affected by oral magnesium preparations.

Magnesium serves as a coenzyme for approximately 80 percent of the enzymes in the body and is the fourth most abundant element in the human body. Researchers believe that magnesium levels may be decreased as a result of stress, anxiety, or low physical activity. A major factor that contributes to magnesium deficiency, however, is a reduction in available dietary magnesium in the diet. There is also a low concentration of magnesium in our water and soil. In addition, there are numerous medical conditions that produce a net loss of magnesium from the body (**Table 15**).

TABLE 15

<u>CAUSES OF MAGNESIUM DEFICIENCY</u>

1. Excessive Urinary Loss Diuretics
   Alcohol abuse
   Diabetic ketoacidosis
   Antibiotics
   Postobstructive diuresis
   Hypercalcemia
   Syndrome of inappropriate antidiuretic hormone secretion

2. Decrease in Intestinal Absorption
   Prolonged gastrointestinal suction
   Surgical resection of bowel
   Diarrheal states
   Various bowel diseases
   H-2 receptor antagonist therapy (Tagamet or Zantac)

3. Decreased Intake
   Alcohol abuse
   Parenteral alimentation IV therapy inadequate in magnesium
   Protein-caloric malnutrition
   Starvation

In the absence of renal disease, magnesium supplements may be taken without fear of adverse reactions. Magnesium chloride is a good choice in that it is well absorbed. *The best sources of magnesium in the diet are sea vegetables, sesame seeds, green leafy vegetables, fish, meat, seafood, brown rice, soybean products, whole grains, bananas, apricots, nuts and seeds* (**Table 16**).

Magnesium also has one other vital protective function in the body. *It helps to counteract aluminum toxicity,* which is gaining increasing popularity in both the medical and lay literature. **Newsweek,** August 1991, published an article on Alzheimer's disease, mentioning its casual relationship to aluminum. More recently, there has been futher evidence suggesting that there is a connection between aluminum toxicity in the environment and its relationship to the lesions in the brain that cause Alzheimer's disease. Like many of the other environmental toxins, the accumulation of aluminum may go on for years, eventually taking its toll on the body.

Aluminum is a toxic metal; unfortunately, it is still being used in drugs, food, particularly junk food, additives, and packaging, as well as pots and pans. Aluminum is also the major component used in our cans. It is found in antacids, foil, deodorants, bleached white flour, and even in our water. Aluminum has no known benefit to the human body. In addition to the possible connection with Alzheimer's disease, aluminum may cause other central nervous system disturbances as well as enhance the process of osteoporosis.

It makes sense to avoid aluminum as much as possible, particularly since the environment is so overwhelmed by it. My recommendation would be to *exchange any aluminum cookware for stainless steel, iron, or glass.*

TABLE 16

FOODS HIGH IN MAGNESIUM

Cereal and Grains	Fruits
All Bran	**Figs, dried
Brown rice	Vegetables
Fish	Adzuki beans
All seafood	Black beans
Nuts and Seeds	Navy beans
**Pumpkin seeds	**Kelp
Sesame seeds	Spinach
Soybean nuts	Wakame
Sunflower seeds	**Tofu
	White beans

(**Foods Highest in Magnesium)

Read labels to avoid compounds containing aluminum. *Eat a diet high in fiber and foods that inhibit aluminum absorption, including almonds, spinach, and rhubarb.* The B vitamins, particularly B-6, are also recommended. In addition to a high-fiber diet, magnesium, calcium, vitamin C, and zinc are helpful nutrients in counteracting aluminum toxicity.

POTASSIUM

Potassium is one mineral that concerns physicians. Drugs for the treatment of high blood pressure or congestive heart failure may interfere with potassium absorption and excretion. The effects of either low potassium or high potassium can be life threatening. Since potassium is necessary for the healthy functioning of nerves, cells, and membranes, it is an important electrolyte to monitor. Low potassium is a major cause of cardiac arrhythmia. Although potassium supplementation is usually not necessary, individuals on diuretics, laxatives, or who have excessive diarrhea may require extra potassium. Caution should be taken, however, in those individuals with renal insufficiency as additional potassium in the diet may not be excreted by the kidney. We should be able to get all the potassium we need from our diet. The highest levels of potassium are found in *sea vegetables, fruits, vegetables, fish, lean meat, poultry, garlic, raisins, bananas, apricots, and whole grains* (**Table 17**). Coffee and alcohol, however, may deplete potassium in the body. Alcohol can deplete the body's magnesium levels as well. When consuming such beverages, it is important to maintain a proper potassium intake.

TABLE 17

FOODS HIGH IN POTASSIUM

Cereals
All Bran
Bran Buds
Raisin Bran

Fruits
Apricots
Bananas
Cantelope

Dates
**Figs
Nectarines
**Prunes, dried
**Raisins

Fish
Anchovies
Bass, fresh water
Bluefish
Catfish
Clams
Crab, Blue
Flounder/Sole
Haddock
Halibut
Lobster
Mackerel
Mussels
Perch
Salmon
Snapper
Swordfish
Trout
Tuna

Milk/Yogurt
Skim milk
Lofat yogurt
Skim yogurt

Nuts and Seeds
**Soybean nuts

Vegetables
**Adzuki Beans
**Avocado
Bamboo Shoots
Beet greens
Black beans
Turtle beans
Chard, Swiss
Chickpeas
French beans
Garlic
Great Northern Beans
Kidney beans
Lentils
**Lima beans
Navy Beans
Pinto beans
Potato with skin
Nori
Natto (soybean product)
Squash, Acorn
Sweet Potato
**White beans

Meats/Poultry
Rib eye
Beef round eye
Goose without skin

(** Foods Highest in Potassium)

Selenium

Selenium is considered a cardiologist's mineral, as it is protective to the heart. Selenium is an active antioxidant and a scavanger of free radicals. It is important to the immune system and has been regarded as an agent in the protection from cancer. For example, cancer and heart disease occur considerably less in the Oriental cultures than in the West. Since the Orient has considerable quantities of selenium in their soils, the Asian diet is rich in selenium. Studies have demonstrated that *people who eat selenium, whether in food or in supplement form, develop less cancers, particularly of the breast, colon, and prostate.* When combined with vitamin E, selenium is a powerful antioxidant and its efficacy is much greater in combination.

Selenium protects against environmental pollutants such as lead and cadmium and is a major antagonist against the toxic effects of mercury, which is prevalent in dental fillings, cosmetics, pesticides, and in saltwater fish, particularly tuna. *Prominent sources of selenium include fish, sea vegetables, whole grains, wheat germ, garlic, onions, chicken, brown rice, and broccoli.* There are no known side effects. The recommended daily maintenance dose of selenium is approximately 50-200 micrograms.

Iron

Iron, in simple terms, is essential for the production of hemoglobin, which is found in red blood cells. Without iron, we would develop anemia. This is the mineral most prevalent in blood. Deficiencies in iron include anemic symptoms such as fatigue, pallor, and dizziness. Other symptoms of iron deficiency include brittle hair, hair loss, and ridging of the nails. Several factors influence the amount of iron absorbed in the diet. A degree of hydrochloric acid (natural stomach acidity) must be present in the stomach in order for iron to be absorbed. Vitamin C can also increase iron absorption by as much as 30 percent. Iron absorption can be decreased by antacids, aspirin, caffeine, and some food preservatives.

The most common cause of iron deficiency results from bleeding, either through the gastrointestinal tract, or through excessive menstrual bleeding. Iron deficiency is more likely to occur in rapidly growing teenagers as well as menstruating women. Iron supplementation is recommended in pregnancy as well as in cases of chronic blood loss. The RDA for iron is approximately 10–18 mg per day. Since we can obtain much of the iron needed from our diet and environment, it is not recommended for healthy men to take iron supplements. Young women, however, could take iron on a daily basis and especially when pregnant. Since iron is stored in the body, excessive iron taken over a considerable period of time can cause problems particularly in the liver, heart, and pancreas. Iron overload, thus, can go unnoticed and can be quite insidious in its onset. Individuals who drink considerable quantities of iron contained in red wine, and in addition, take iron supplements, may develop headache, shortness of breath, and easy fatiguability, symptoms of iron overload. Iron cookware is yet another source where one can obtain additional amounts of iron from the environment.

The best sources of iron include sea vegetables, green leafy vegetables, whole grains, lean meats, eggs, poultry, dates, beans, lentils, parsley peaches, raisins, rice, dried fruits, molasses, and sesame seeds.

IODINE

Iodine is especially important in the healthy functioning of the thyroid gland. It calms the body and relieves nervous tension. Although it is only needed in trace amounts, iodine deficiencies may occur, particularly if drinking water is chlorinated. If this is the case, and if too little iodine is taken into the diet, nervous and mental deficiencies may occur. One may have the inability to think clearly. Irritability and difficulty sleeping may be symptoms of iodine deficiency. Iodine deficiency may also occur in soils that are not ladenwith iodine. The best sources of iodine include *sea vegetables, saltwater fish, Swiss chard, watercress, turnip greens, mushrooms, bananas, cabbage, and onions.*

TABLE 18

FOODS HIGH IN IRON

Cereals and Grains	Miscellaneous
Oatmeal	Eggs
Bran Buds	**Vegetables**
Bran Flakes	Artichokes
Product 19	Turtle beans
Brown rice	Chickpeas
Fish	Great Northern beans
Clams	Kidney beans
Oysters	**Lentils
Fruits	Lima beans
**Figs, dried	Navy beans
Peaches	**Tofu
Prunes, dried	Spinach
Dates	**White beans
Raisins	**Meat**
Nuts and Seeds	Liver, beef
Sesame seeds	Liver, Chicken
Pumpkin seeds, dried	Liver, Turkey

(**Foods Highest in Iron)

MINERALS AND YOU

There are many important minerals that the body utilizes in normal functioning. Many of these are trace elements that are extremely useful in preserving the health and everyday maintenance of the body, sometimes referred by doctors as homeostasis. At the time I was writing this book, I had the opportunity of visiting a chemical laboratory where vitamins were produced. I learned from the chemists on staff that the FDA would come into the laboratory from time to time and check for quality control. After going on a tour through the factory and seeing the way vitamins and minerals were made, I was impressed by the complexity of their formulas. Meticulous arrangements for the preparation of various formulas could be created for both healthy and unhealthy populations alike. For instance, many of us need to take potassium, magnesium, and manganese on a daily basis. However, in an individual with renal insufficiency, potassium needs to be limited. Thus, it is important to choose the right vitamin and mineral preparations. Many such combinations may contain copper and iron as well. Although copper is needed to make red blood cells, we tend to get all the copper we need from the environment, as it is frequently found in our drinking water. Iron is yet another element that is also plentiful in the environment. Some vitamin manufacturers do not place excess iron in their formulas because of its pro-oxidant properties. Unfortunately, many multi-vitamins and mineral preparations do include, in my opinion, excess quantities of iron and copper. Naturally, if iron supplementation is required for iron deficiency anemia or in menstruating young women, then it could be utilized without any undue side effects. However, since iron is stored in the body and accumulates over time, this is one mineral that should not be consumed in doses greater than the RDA which is essentially 10-18 mg.

The RDA for copper is 2 mg, and frequently, multi-vitamin and mineral preparations will include both copper and iron in their formulas. Although I am not recommending that we stay away from such formulas, we need to keep in mind that over consumption of copper and iron could exist. Therefore, it is my recommendation that we choose vitamin and mineral formulas that contain equal or less than the RDA requirements. In the following examples of mineral, vitamin/antioxidant formulas, you will see that I suggested minimal iron and one-quarter of the RDA for copper. The reader will also note that the fat soluble vitamins, i.e. A, D, and E, are not represented in very large doses. Here again, since these vitamins are taken on a daily basis and are stored in the body, high doses of these nutrients are not recommended. The following vitamin and mineral formulas are similar to what I am presently taking. If I were to devise a formula, I would include the following ingredients (see tables). Again, the reader has to realize that this vitamin and mineral formula is not for everyone. For example, the potassium content in this formula would be considered too high for individuals with renal insufficiency. Likewise, if an individual forms calcium stones in the urine, the amount of calcium in this formula would also be excessive. Generally speaking, however, the enclosed formulas, with minor exceptions, would suit the needs of most people. For selected individuals, additional nutritional supplements may be helpful in weight loss management. Here again, the reader will see that *vitamin B-6, Q_{10}, zinc, chromium picolinate, and GTF could be considered additional supplements to the already suggested vitamin and mineral formulas.* There is also some evidence to suggest that *kelp, garlic, parsley, fennel, spirulina, Glucomannan, and various amino acids, especially L–Carnitine, may also aid in fat digestion and weight management as well.*

The reader needs to keep in mind, however, that supplements only serve as additional therapy to a well-balanced, nutritious, high-fiber, low-fat program. Many of these vitamin and nutritional supplements can be purchased in health food stores. It is important to understand, however, that it really isn't vitamins, minerals or nutritional supplements like bee pollen, or green barley malt, or a cookie, or whatever new panacea becomes popular that will make the difference in our lives. But using such supplements and high-fiber, low-fat foods is a place to start. From this place, we can branch out to other health healing foods and truly change our dietary lifestyles, and thereby change our emotional and physical health. Awareness, once again, is the key to healing.

TABLE 19

MINERAL ANTIOXIDANT FORMULA
DOSE – 2 CAPTABS/DAY

FORMULA/CAPTAB:

Calcium	600 mg
Potassium	99 mg
Magnesium	300 mg
Manganese	3 mg
Zinc	15 mg
Vanadium	0.1 ppm
Chromium (GTF)	100 mcg
Iodine	75 mcg
Selenium	100 mcg
Molybdenum	100 mcg
Boron	1.5 mg
Silicon	Trace
Iron	1.8 mg
Copper	0.5 mg
L-Cysteine	125 mcg
L-Methionine	50 mg
L-Glutathione	15 mg

TABLE 20

VITAMIN ANTIOXIDANT FORMULA

DOSE – 2 CAPTABS/DAY

FORMULA/CAPTAB:

Vitamin A (palmatate)	1,000 I.U.
Beta-Carotene (pro vitamin A)	5,000 I.U.
Vitamin D	200 I.U.
Vitamin C	250 mg
Vitamin E	200 I.U.
Bioflavonoid Complex	100 mg
Vitamin B-1	18.75 mg
Vitamin B-2	18.75 mg
Vitamin B-6	18.75 mg
Vitamin B-3 (niacinamide)	50 mg
Vitamin B-12	50 mg
Vitamin B-5 (panothenic acid)	50 mg
Folic Acid	200 mcg
PABA	18.75 mg
Biotin	200 mg
Choline Bitartrate	50 mg
Inositol	25 mg

TABLE 21

ADDITIONAL NUTRITIONAL SUPPLEMENTS FOR WEIGHT LOSS

DOSE – 2 CAPTABS/DAY

FORMULA/CAPTAB:

Coenzyme Q_{10}	15 mg
Zinc	10 mg
Vitamin B-6	18.75 mg
L-Carnitine	50 mcg
Chromium (GTF)	100 mcg

135

CHAPTER 11

FOODS THAT HEAL

This is a chapter about nutritional awareness. A prudent diet is your best asset in weight reduction and your best defense against illness. Nutritional healing utilizes a diet that makes you feel better both in body and mind. The old cliche "you are what you eat" is basically true. This chapter is designed to look at foods that enhance and nourish your body. We have previously discussed the advantages of complex carbohydrates, monounsaturated fats, the importance of water, along with various vitamins and minerals, and the negative aspects of both caffeine and alcohol. This chapter is about taking on a new array of foods. In the spirit on nondeprivation, and with the slow and patient approach, we can learn to use less of certain foods and more of new ones that can be equally enjoyable.

Changing your food patterns may not be easy. Since you have been building your eating habits all of your life, it may be difficult to substitute one type of food for another. But with an open mind, it doesn't have to be painful. On the contrary, experimenting with new recipes and foodstuffs can be fun. For example, for years I loved red meat. I then gradually switched to chicken and fish for most of my animal protein and enjoy my food as much as ever. The transition to a healthier diet may take some time. *My first exposure to seaweed was a disaster!* It tasted too fishy and I didn't like it. Gradually it became palatable, and now I find it most enjoyable. During the transition phase I would recommend you gradually do the following:

1. Reduce the amount of red meat in the diet.
2. Reduce dairy products, particularly whole milk and high fat cheeses and ice creams.
3. Reduce eggs.
4. Reduce saturated fats.
5. Omit refined sugars including white table sugar.
6. Reduce refined flour and bleached flours.
7. Omit as much processed food as possible.
8. Limit sodium intake.
9. Reduce alcohol consumption and caffeine intake.
10. Increase fiber consumption.
11. Increase complex carbohydrates in terms of whole grains, pastas, and beans.
12. Increase consumption of fresh fruits and vegetables.
13. Increase consumption of sea vegetables.

Most expert nutritionists and some physicians, particularly those interested in a macrobiotic approach, feel that an optimal diet should include approximately 40 percent whole grains. Whole grains (wheat, corn, rice, oats, millet, rye, barley, and buckwheat) are those that are unrefined and are exceedingly nutritious. They contain more vitamins, minerals, and fiber than their lighter, whiter, and fluffier counterparts found in commercially packaged goods. In their raw form, grains contain a seed and a covering to protect the seed. With the advent of the Industrial Revolution and modern processing, it became easier to remove the germ and bran layers, making available to the general population white flours that were once reserved only for the rich.

Unfortunately, these discarded segments contain all the fiber and the vast majority of the B-complex vitamins, as well as the vitamins E and A and the minerals magnesium, potassium, zinc, iron, and selenium. In refining grains, the flour is commonly bleached, giving it a lighter, seemingly more presentable image and a softer texture. Additionally, these refined grains are frequently laced with additives and preservatives. White flour used in white bread and pastries contains many empty calories. It provides carbohydrates, but little fiber. Most of the carbohydrates are not eliminated, but rather converted to glucose and stored as fats in the body.

With greater awareness, many people are now purchasing breads that favor a whole-grain concept. Wheat breads and fiber breads are now quite plentiful in supermarkets, but *the best source of vitamins and minerals and fiber found in whole-grain bread products are those available from your local health food store or bakery.* Since whole grain is unrefined and contains multiple nutrients, this is the closest thing to a complete food because it contains not only carbohydrates, but also a balanced amount of protein, low fats, and multiple vitamins and minerals and sufficient fiber.

Civilizations all over the world have been utilizing grain for centuries as a diet staple. Primitive cultures are also known to have the lowest prevalence rates of cancer and heart disease. Grains, as we discussed in an earlier analysis, decrease the transitory time of waste through the bowel and in addition to having high fiber, also are made up of polysaccharides. These complex sugars are less quickly converted to glucose than simple sugars found in refined products, therefore, less available for conversion to fat. It is important to incorporate whole grains in your diet, and it would be my recommendation to intake one to two servings per day. The following is a list of good possible grains.

BROWN RICE – Brown rice may be obtained in the short, medium, or long grain varieties. It is also available in a sweet version called Basmati. In addition to containing many of the vitamins and minerals mentioned, brown rice contains the mineral silicon, which is a necessary element for our body. Some investigators point out that silicon helps prevent "burn-out" in high performance individuals who drive themselves excessively in both their personal and professional lives. Brown rice is easy to cook. It can be boiled, steamed, or even fried. To cook brown rice, wash the grain thoroughly and soak it in water for several minutes; rinse and drain; add one cup of grain to two cups of water and a pinch of salt in a sauce pan; bring to a boil; immediately cover the pot and turn down the heat to simmer; do not lift the lid or stir until the water has been absorbed, approximately 45-50 minutes. This is the way I prefer to cook brown rice. I frequently will cook two cups of rice at a time and then reheat it for use over the next few days. Brown rice is an excellent complex carbohydrate that goes well with almost any fish dish. When brown rice is used in combination with beans, it provides excellent sources of protein in the diet.

BARLEY – Barley is grown throughout the world and is a popular grain in America. It is chewy and has a nutty taste. Barley has been used as a natural sweetener and in making beer. It is an excellent grain to use in soups or it can be mixed with brown rice and served as a side dish. Merely add one-third cup of barley to one cup of brown rice and prepare in the same manner as brown rice.

BUCKWHEAT – Buckwheat is technically the seed of a fruit rather than a true grain. It has a rich and somewhat bitter flavor. The Eastern cultures grind buckwheat into flour to create noodles. It is a good flour to use, particularly in pancakes. A pancake recipe is included in this text.

MILLET – Millet is a grain that was used traditionally for centuries by the peoples of Africa and China. Millet can be boiled by itself or with a variety of vegetables. It goes especially well with broccoli or cauliflower and may be substituted for brown rice or barley.

CORN – For centuries, corn has been the stable grain of the Indian cultures in North and Central America. It is frequently not considered a grain, but it actually is. Corn can be ground into flour to make cornmeal, which may be used to make cereals, polenta, and tortillas. It also makes a delicious muffin. This is an excellent substitute for people allergic to wheat. Whole corn or corn-on-the-cob contains good sources of fiber as well as vitamins and minerals, particularly beta carotene.

WHEAT – Wheat is especially rich in B vitamins and vitamin E. In its refined form, it is lacking many of the important nutrients, but in the form of whole-wheat flour or berries, it provides excellent sources of minerals and vitamins. Wheat berries, when cooked, create a tasty and nutritious dish with a hearty, chewy texture.

Other grains that can be consumed include *oats, rye, and wild rice.* Any of these grains are strongly recommended. Another highly nutritious food that I recommend to many of my clients is *Soba, or the buckwheat noodles of Japan.* They are frequently used in soups but may be used as a pasta. *Pasta,* in my opinion, is one of the best foods we can consume. Not only does it taste good, but it is low in fat and contains coarse carbohydrates. It is also easy to prepare and goes well with a numerous variety of sauces, vegetables, meats and fishes. I recommend my cardiovascular clients to eat either pasta or rice on a daily basis.

COMMERCIAL FOR CARLA'S PASTA

In Chapter 12, I'll share several of the recipes that I personally use to prepare my pasta dishes. Like whole grains, pasta can be prepared in many different ways and in many styles. The herbs and spices that may accompany pasta, i.e., *basil, garlic, onions, and parsley,* are magnificent ingredients that have a healing quality on the body, particularly the heart. Dry packaged pasta, either in its traditional form made with *semolina flour* or made from *whole-wheat flours* is an excellent high complex carbohydrate. Fresh or frozen pasta, however, contains eggs. Fortunately, one manufacturer I asked has been able to make a fresh frozen pasta with minimal egg yolk. Usually, it takes six eggs to make one pound of fresh frozen pasta, which is greater than 1200 mg of cholesterol per pound. *Carla's Pasta* in Manchester, Connecticut, offers a fresh frozen pasta made from predominately egg whites with only one egg yolk instead of six. It can be shipped and stored and has greater than 90 percent of the fat and cholesterol removed.

MORE RECOMMENDATIONS FOR HEALING FOODS

In this analysis, we have discussed whole grains and pastas as being healing foods in our diet. Another highly nutritious food that I would recommend even on a daily basis is *beans.* Beans are high in calcium and contain twice as much protein in comparable volumes as meat and poultry or dairy food. When combined with grains, they provide all the needed essential amino acids. They are really the best single vegetarian source of protein. Some bean products include *black-eyed peas, chick-peas, lentils, pinto beans, split peas, adzuki, and lima beans.* Any of these bean combinations are good. Lentils are a particular favorite of mine, especially in soups. They are easy to digest as well as to prepare, and they also provide an excellent source of vegetable iron. Boiling is perhaps the best method for cooking beans. Frequently, they should be soaked overnight. When boiled, a pinch of salt and/or stalk of seaweed may be added. Cooking usually takes between one and one-half and two hours. Like short-grained brown rice, beans can be cooked and reheated for later use.

Soybeans are perhaps the highest in protein and are a favorite in macrobiotic cooking. *Tofu, tempeh, tamari, and miso* are all made from soybeans and are easily found in health food stores. Miso is a particular favorite of mine, and in its soup form is highly recommended to virtually all clients in our weight-reducing program as well as many of my heart patients. Miso is made from fermented soybeans, grains, and seasalt, and contains many of the enzymes that strengthen the body.

In a major Japanese study, *those who ate miso soup every day had a significantly lower risk of dying from cancer and heart disease compared to those who never consumed miso or only on occasion.* This large prospective study, in excess of over a quarter of a million people, demonstrates one of the best kept secrets of Oriental medicine. Based on my review of the medical literature, particularly with the overwhelming evidence of population studies, it appears that sea vegetables and the miso preparations do enhance health and longevity. Miso is used in the recipe for sea vegetable soup that follows in the chapter *Recipes For Life.*

The next section of this chapter will include particular foods that I feel have healing properties. For example, we briefly discussed *sea vegetables,* which were reported in lowering heart disease in Japan. The highest incidence of longevity is found in the village of Oki on Oki Island, whose inhabitants eat large amounts of sea vegetables. Compared with other regions of Japan, these villages also have an unusually low rate of stroke. I prefer sea vegetables not only because of the high vitamin and nutritional constituents, but also because they are protective against minor effects of nuclear radioactivity. Medical research has determined that sea vegetables contain a substance called sodium alginate that helps eliminate from the body radioactive strontium, a breakdown product of uranium. As we intake minute amounts of radiation from sources as various as the sun to x-rays and microwaves, sea vegetables are a good form of insurance.

Sea Vegetables

My first introduction to sea vegetables resulted from the use of miso soup. After some minor research, in which I learned that sea vegetables are highly nutritious and help eliminate unwanted fats in our bodies, I decided to use them in our weight-reducing program. After making several types of miso soups with the various combinations, I experimented with *wakame* and *kombu seaweeds*. My first exposure to these seaweeds was not good; I found them distasteful and very "fishy." Nevertheless, because of their nutritional value, I put minor elements of the seaweeds in the soups. Some of my patients, however, really savored the taste. As a matter of fact, in our group support sessions, I was amazed to see how many of the people really thoroughly enjoyed these miso soup preparations. Yet, I wasn't sold on the taste.

It wasn't until my sister came to my house and made a sea vegetable soup that I learned how versatile they really are. She had recently undergone a hysterectomy and received considerable doses of radiation to the pelvis and abdomen. Because of her interest in reducing the effects of radiation, she bought Schechter's book on food and radiation. In the book she found a recipe for "Sea Vegetable Soup." To say this soup was delicious would be an understatement. It was outstanding! I have altered this recipe only slightly. After consuming the sea vegetable soup on several occasions, I developed a particular affinity for it. The combination of the vegetable oil, miso, and the herbs of thyme and marjoram made this a very flavorful and satisfying concoction. I actually felt better after I consumed this soup. I had more energy. I felt more alive and became more clear. It wasn't just a coincidence, either. *I really believe in the "healing" properties of this broth.*

Since the time of recorded history, seaweeds have been utilized by many cultures in various portions of the world. They have been harvested from the coastal waters of Japan, Ireland, France, and Canada. In our own country, for example, they have been taken from the Maine coastal waters. After doing considerable research into seaweeds, I became convinced that they have both a protective and a healing effect on the body. Sea vegetables are extremely rich in vitamins, minerals, and nutrients. In fact, *they contain all 56 minerals!* As a group of foods, sea vegetables contain the highest amounts of magnesium, iron, iodine, and sodium. For those individuals who have a history of congestive heart failure or high blood pressure, it is recommended that sea vegetables be consumed only one time per week. It is also important to soak seaweeds for at least one-half hour before preparation. By soaking them in tap water or spring water, the sodium content will be reduced.

As seaweeds contain extremely high amounts of calcium and phosphorous, they would be beneficial in situations where calcium is needed in the body, such as osteoporosis. They are also approximately 25 percent protein and two percent fat. They are low in calories, which makes them an extremely useful adjunct to diet therapy where one wants to limit calories from fats. Seaweeds are rich in many trace elements, as well. For example, they are high in beta carotene, vitamin B-12, niacin, pantothenic acid (B-5), and vitamins A, C, and E, as well as the mineral selenium. Selenium, combined with vitamins A, C, and E, and beta carotene, is extremely important in the overall functioning of the heart. In the Chinese culture, where the incidence of heart disease is markedly lower, selenium is found in the soil. Some investigators believe that it is the intake of selenium that offers a protective environment for the healthy functioning of the heart.

In summary, many clinical studies indicate that seaweed is one of nature's best nutritional supplements in healing. It contains virtually all of the minerals and vitamins that are useful in preventing "free radical formation." Sea vegetables have been utilized in treating cancer, lowering blood cholesterol, thinning the blood, and even preventing ulcers. Sea vegetables are also known for their effect on dissolving fat deposits and eliminating heavy metal contaminants from the body, including radiation, cadmium, and other environmental toxins. Oriental folklore and fact show that consumption of sea vegetables offers a nutritional package that is simple, inexpensive, and easy to prepare. It is a dietary supplement that should be used by everyone. Seaweed is one of nature's wonders!

VEGETABLES

Although some of my macrobiotic colleagues may disagree, I believe that most vegetables are healthful to our bodies. My only restriction at this point includes *avocado* and *olives. Avocado and olives contain abundant sources of fat,* and olives contain considerable quantities of sodium as well. Most vegetables contain an abundant source of vitamins, including beta carotene. I do have a preference for *organically grown vegetables.* Remember that organic vegetables are not cultivated with pesticides, herbicides, or fertilizers. *Vegetables should make up approxi-*

mately 25-40 percent of the calories in our diet, including leafy green, round, and root vegetables. For example, daikon, a root vegetable resembling a long white radish, has a high calcium content and is extremely useful in healing. We have recommended the use of daikon in some of our miso soup preparations. Roots are also rich in complex carbohydrates as well as vitamins and minerals. *Carrots* and *parsnips* are excellent root vegetables to consume. In general, most of the "non starchy" vegetables from asparagus to zucchini contain approximately two grams of protein and five grams of carbohydrate per one-half cup serving. The more starchy vegetables such as corn-on-the-cob, lima beans or potatoes, have approximately 15 grams of carbohydrate and two grams of protein per one-half cup serving. Vegetables make excellent choices in our diet.

Green vegetables including cabbage, kale, leeks, broccoli, watercress, brussels sprouts, parsley, turnip greens, and bok choy offer tremendous sources of vitamins A and C. Kale, for example, is abundant in calcium, yielding approximately 300 mg per cup, which is similar to four ounces of daikon or a cup of milk. Remember that vegetables contain no cholesterol and are virtually free of fat. They are also rich in fiber and easy to digest.

The round vegetables include *turnips, cabbage, pumpkins, potatoes, beets, garlic, and onions, to mention a few.* As a cardiologist, I am particularly interested in garlic and onions, about which I will go into further detail later.

Vegetables can be cooked in many ways such as boiling, steaming, stir frying, baking, or pressure cooking as well as simmering them in stews and soups. *Raw vegetables are preferred when possible, especially with the skins intact.*

Almost every vegetable is good for you. Some have particular advantages. *Turnips* are exceedingly high in vitamin A, for example. *Artichokes* are abundant in iron and *asparagus* is high in chlorophyll. Chlorophyll, found in the tops of vegetables, alfalfa sprouts, and green leaves, contains an abundance of iron and is a tremendous red cell builder. If you prefer lettuce, try *leaf lettuce* over iceberg head lettuce. Leaf lettuce has almost as much as a hundred times of iron as head lettuce. You really can't go wrong by consuming as many vegetables as possible. The list is endless and far beyond the scope of this text. The reader is encouraged to try as many vegetables as desired.

FRUITS

Most fruits contain potassium and vitamin C. As a clinical cardiologist, I prefer my clients to ingest one to two servings of fruit a day, especially if on diuretics, which deplete potassium. Even though fruits are high in natural sugars that eventually turn into glucose, they also contain abundant sources of fiber, as well as beta carotene and pectin. *Grapefruit* is the highest in pectin, and from a previous analysis, we know that pectin yields a favorable blood cholesterol profile. In an article in **Cardiology World News,** September 1991, animal research indicates that pectin may not only reduce cholesterol, but also may lower the incidence of cancer. It was demonstrated that grapefruit pectin, even in the face of a high fat diet, restricted the development of atherosclerosis. It is important to remember to eat fruits in their fresh state. Fruits grown locally and in season are the best. Dried fruits also need to be considered. I frequently recommend my clients *eat dates, currants, raisins, and figs one to two times a week.* Again, though they are high in natural sugar, they are a source of calcium as well as vitamins and fiber.

SEEDS AND NUTS

Although a small amount of seeds and nuts may provide a crunchy and tasty part of the diet, most contain high quantities of saturated fat. Most of the calories in peanut butter, for example, are derived from fat. It is my recommendation that *peanut butter be strictly avoided in all diets but those of growing children. Walnuts also contain approximately 80 percent fat.* Almonds, on the other hand, are more favorable, and in some clinical studies have been shown to improve cholesterol levels. *Chestnuts* are the lowest in fat and are good eaten raw or roasted. *Sesame seeds,* although containing some fat, are exceedingly high in vitamins C and E, as well as calcium and protein. Toasted sesame may be ground as an exceptional condiment called tahini, which can be used in salad dressings and soups. Tahini can be purchased at health food stores or in some supermarkets. Remember, the unhulled seeds have a longer shelf life than hulled seeds, which are more prone to spoilage after losing their protective coating.

SOUPS

Soups can be made with a wide variety of vegetables, beans, grains, and particularly sea vegetables. Keep in mind that sea vegetables, especially *kelp,* is exceedingly abundant in magnesium and has 150 times more iodine than any of the commonly used land vegetables. Soups are also another way to incorporate *Shitake* (Shi-tah-kee) *mushrooms* in our diets. These Japanese mushrooms have been used for centuries as an ancient Oriental medicine said to promote vitality and youth. As studies have shown, they build resistance against viruses and have been used in the treatment of some cancers. They have also been used to treat fatigue. When preparing the dry Shitake mushrooms, it is best to cut them up into small pieces and place them in soups. They have a distinct flavor and can be easily assimilated into the diet. Try incorporating more soup into your diet for a low-calorie way of obtaining healthy vitamins and minerals.

SWEETENERS

As we have seen in the previous analysis, *the use of table sugar should be strictly avoided* in the diet. Other natural sweeteners are preferred. For example, *barley malt, rice syrup, and apple juice* make excellent sweeteners. Although I may be going out on a limb, I will recommend *honey.* Some of my colleagues may have difficulty with this recommendation, but after much research and scrutiny into honey, I do believe this is an acceptable food that we need to consider in our diets. Since honey contains several amino acids and large amounts of B-complex vitamins as well as C, D, E, and minerals, honey is not considered an empty-calorie food as sugar is. And because it is twice as sweet as most other sugars, smaller amounts can be used.

Honey comes from the nectar of flowers which is collected in the bee's honey sac. One tiny worker bee is known to produce approximately one-half teaspoon of honey during its lifetime. Honey occurs naturally and is not produced artificially. It is made up of water, dextrose, levulose, and other substances, including resins, gums, and pollen. The therapeutic uses of honey as a healing agent have been passed on by multiple civilizations over the ages. Honey is an outstanding energy food. I remember our coaches telling us to swallow honey prior to our athletic bouts. It is a far better sweetener than monosaccharides such as glucose, and it doesn't require additional metabolic energy to digest.

Honey has also been used as a remedy in hay fever, allergies, sleep disorders, and fighting sore throats and colds. I am particularly impressed with Dr. Jarvis' Vermont Folk Medicine in which he discusses the therapeutic and healing effects of honey. I have tried some of his recommendations on myself, such as his cold remedy of one tablespoon of honey and one tablespoon of apple cider vinegar with four ounces of warm water. I found it quite nurturing and healing. Since honey quickly enters the blood, however, it needs to be utilized with caution by diabetics. Because honey is a raw food, it also should not be given to infants as their immune systems are not fully developed.

Another food related to honey is *bee pollen* which, like honey, contains an abundance of vitamins and nutrients. The human consumption of bee pollen dates back to antiquity and was frequently used in the Olympic games in Greece. Now in the 20th Century, bee pollen is gaining increasing popularity as being effective protection against many of the common pollutants in the environment including carbon monoxide, lead, mercury, and nitrites. Bee pollen is used in the treatment of allergies, similar to an allergy shot, as it desensitizes the individual. There have also been studies showing that bee pollen strengthens the resistance of immune systems in both cancer and radiation studies. This is one particular product that may become more popular because of its nutritional and high protein values.

GARLIC AND ONIONS

Garlic and onions are considered by cardiologists to be some of the most healing foods. Many clinical studies show that garlic and onions contain an active anticoagulant that acts very similar to aspirin. Garlic has been know to lower blood pressure and inhibit platelet aggregation, thus reducing the possibility of blood clotting. Garlic and onions also can lower LDL cholesterol and raise the beneficial HDL cholesterol levels as well. I recommend both *raw onions* and *lightly cooked onions* to my patients. There have been several worldwide clinical studies to show the beneficial metabolic and blood-clotting effects of garlic and onions. In addition to the favorable cardiological effects, garlic has been touted as a potent immune system stimulant. Since garlic contains sulfa-like compounds, it is a natural antibiotic. When garlic is crushed, the compound Allicin in formed. Allicin is a sulfur compound capable of killing 23 kinds of bacteria including Salmonella and at least sixty types of fungi and yeasts, including Candida.

Garlic and onions constitute a major portion of my diet as I frequently use them in many of my sauces and salad dressings. Garlic is great to use with fish, particularly when marinating. It works well with swordfish, bluefish, and flounder. For example, I will frequently marinate a fish with a dressing of chopped garlic, small amounts of white wine, freshly squeezed lemon, and freshly ground basil with one to two tablespoons of olive oil. Pour this over fish and sprinkle with fresh parsley. Marinate in the refrigerator for several hours or perhaps overnight. This type of marinade works well to take the "fishy taste" out of bluefish. When cooking, garlic can be chopped into fine pieces or can be used as whole cloves. The major drawback to garlic is the odor, but if you are concerned about the odor, eating parsley after garlic or chewing on fennel will help alleviate the aftertaste and odors. *My recommendations for utilizing garlic and onions would be to eat them as much as possible.* The only major problem with overuse is upset stomach and occasional allergic reaction.

PARSLEY

You are probably wondering why I recommend garnishing with parsley in most of my recipes. Parsley contains a high concentration of chlorophyll, which is similar to the red blood cell structure called hemoglobin. Parsley is an excellent vegetable protein and in addition to chlorophyll, contains high quantities of iron as well as vitamins A, and C. It is also interesting to note that chlorophyll combats the effects of radiation in experimental animal studies. This may be why it is considered an anti-cancer agent. Fresh parsley not only tastes great, but it also yields a beautiful green color to freshly prepared foods, and green is the color associated with good health. Parsley, as well as several other food supplements, does enhance healing.

It is beyond the scope of this text to list the numerous other natural and health/healing ingredients. In addition to the previous books mentioned, I would also endorse Dr. Dean Ornish's *Program for Reversing Heart Disease* and *Prescription for Nutritional Healing by Balch and Balch*. These texts, in my opinion, offer the reader a comprehensive and in-depth approach to natural nutritional awareness and healing.

CHAPTER 12

RECIPES FOR LIFE

The following recipes that you are about to consider are recipes that I use in my daily life. After graduating college in 1968, I managed to keep my weight within 10 to 15 of my wrestling class of 147 pounds. I now weigh 154 pounds. Over the years my diet has mainly been of a Mediterranean nature. For example, I eat *rice* and *pasta* often—I really could eat pasta every day—and I use *whole grains, breads, soups,* and *vegetable stews* as a staple in my diet. The pasta recipes are, for the most part, my own creation. When I don't have pasta, I usually have *brown rice.* I seldom eat red meat and infrequently have chicken or turkey. For the most part, I try to have *fish* at least one to two times a week.

I usually accompany my meals with a simple salad of *lettuce* and tomatoes or *vegetables* marinated in olive oil. I am, however, not perfect. I do "indulge" now and then and eat less healthy foods when they are prepared for me by someone else (a friend, restaurant, party, etc.). I enjoy them too. My point here is that I have discovered ways to eat healthy foods more often and unhealthy foods less often without feeling deprived.

In the following recipes, the frequent use of olive oil is noted. Although it is best to use as little oil as possible, I wholeheartedly endorse the use of olive oil for salads and cooking. Since many of the recipes require two tablespoons of olive oil and most of the recipes are for a family of four or five, the grams of fat per person is still quite reasonable. For example, two tablespoons of olive oil having 28 grams of fat divided by four people would be seven grams of fat, the equivalent of a large tablespoon of ice cream. Even though there are seven grams of fat in the olive oil, the grams of fat in the other constituents are quite low, yielding recipes that are low fat and in most instances, high fiber.

Whenever possible, use fresh ingredients when preparing food, particularly *lemons, basil, parsley, watercress,* and lots of *garlic* and *onions,* all of which are heart-healing. Try to steam as many items as you can. When cooking with oil, use *low heat* and *short cooking times* to prevent "over cooking and oxidation" of oil. Always try to minimize the use of salt and pepper.

MISO SOUP

INGREDIENTS

1 tablespoon toasted Sesame seed oil

2 quarts of water

2 onions, chopped

4 carrots, sliced

2 inches of daikon (Japanese white radish)

1 clove garlic, crushed

10-15 mushrooms, cut in half

4 teaspoons of miso

½ cup of cooked, short-grained brown rice, barley, or uncooked lentils, peas, millet, wheatberries, or adzuki beans

Seasalt and freshly ground pepper

Fresh parsley, or optional watercress or scallions, chopped

DIRECTIONS

Bring water to boil and add chopped onions, carrots, daikon; cover and simmer until vegetables are tender. Add mushrooms which have been sauteed gently in sesame seed oil. Add the miso and simmer for approximately 5-10 minutes. Do not boil. You may wish to add minimal freshly ground pepper and seasalt to taste, one bay leaf and a dash of sesame or olive oil. *You may be creative!* For example, you may add kale, string beans, spinach, or other vegetables. Add one-half cup of cooked rice or other grains of beans. Garnish with freshly chopped parsley, scallions or watercress.

Sea Vegetable Soup - Nature's Wonder

Ingredients

1 cup various sea vegetables (dulse, kelp, wakame, kombu, etc.)

2 quarts spring water

3 tablespooons toasted sesame seed oil

1 large onion, chopped

1 carrot, chopped

1 ½ cups broccoli, chopped

2 cloves garlic, minced

1 teaspoon thyme

1 teaspoon marjoram

Dash of cayenne pepper, freshly ground pepper, or ginger

2 tablespoons miso

Fresh parsley, chopped

Optional ingredients: mushrooms, potatoes, brown rice

Directions

Soak sea vegetables for 30 minutes and discard water (this takes out the excess sodium). Now place in spring water and simmer. Saute onion, carrot, broccoli, and garlic for five minutes, or until onions are partially translucent. Add vegetables to spring water with remaining ingredients, except miso. Simmer for 30 minutes. Turn off heat. Remove ½ cup of liquid and dissolve miso in it. Return to soup and heat for three minutes, do not boil. Adjust seasonings to taste. Garnish with parsley.

This recipe, with slight modification, was taken from *Fighting Radiation with Foods, Herbs, and Vitamins—Documented Natural Remedies that Boost Your Immunity & Detoxify* (Vitality, Inc., 1990), by Steven R. Schechter.

ANTIGUAN BLACK BEAN SOUP

INGREDIENTS

2 tablespoons olive oil

½ green pepper, chopped

1 onion, chopped

½ clove garlic, minced

½ pound dried black beans cooked according to package
   directions or substitute 2 one pound cans of black beans

6 cups water

Fresh ground pepper

2 tablespoons red wine vinegar

1 dried bay leaf

1 cup short-grain brown rice (see brown rice recipe)

Fresh parsley, chopped

DIRECTIONS

In large saucepan, combine olive oil, green pepper, onion, and garlic. Saute' until tender.

Add precooked or canned black beans to six cups of water. Add remaining ingredients and simmer for 30 to 40 minutes with bay leaf. Remove bay leaf before serving and top with chopped onion, short-grain brown rice, or both. Garnish with chopped parsley.

BEET SALAD WITH LEMON AND HONEY

INGREDIENTS

3 medium beets

2 tablespoons olive oil

2 tablespoons red wine vinegar

¼ cup fresh squeezed lemon juice

1 tablespoon honey

1 teaspoon tamari

Fresh chopped parsley

DIRECTIONS

Peel and chop the fresh medium-sized beets into fine pieces, or use a food processor if desired. Make the dressing by first combining the olive oil and red wine vinegar. Add the lemon, honey, and tamari to this and stir briskly. Pour over beets and toss. Sprinkle with freshly chopped parsley.

BOSTON LETTUCE AND WATERCRESS SALAD

INGREDIENTS

1 head Boston lettuce

1 bunch watercress

1 teaspoon whole grain mustard

Seasalt and fresh ground pepper

2 teaspoons finely chopped garlic

1 tablespoon red wine vinegar

½ tablespoon balsamic vinegar

2 tablespoons extra virgin olive oil

Fresh parsley

DIRECTIONS

Remove the core of the lettuce, pull the leaves apart. Cut off the tough ends of the watercress, rinse greens well, and pat dry.

Put the mustard in a salad bowl with salt and pepper. Add the garlic and vinegar and beat with a wire whisk. Gradually add the oil, beating briskly with the wire whisk until well blended. Add the lettuce and watercress. Toss well and serve. Garnish with parsley if desired.

DAD'S ITALIAN STYLE TOMATOES

INGREDIENTS

1 tablespoon olive oil

4 medium to large tomatoes

1 clove garlic, finely chopped

1 tablespoon Balsamic vinegar

Seasalt and freshly ground pepper

Fresh basil or crushed oregano to taste

DIRECTIONS

Wash and dry tomatoes and place in the refrigerator to chill. Slice tomatoes into ¼ inch pieces and place on a plate. Sprinkle drops of olive oil, pieces of garlic, balsamic vinegar, salt, and pepper over the tomatoes. Sprinkle with freshly chopped basil or crushed oregano, but do not use both oregano and basil together.

EASY ITALIAN STYLE TOMATO SAUCE

INGREDIENTS

2 tablespoons olive oil

3 cloves garlic, chopped fine

2 medium onions

2 cans Italian style plum tomatoes, or

2 pounds fresh plum or cherry tomatoes

1 ounce red or white wine

1 tablespoon freshly chopped basil

1 teaspoon freshly crushed oregano

Seasalt and freshly ground pepper

Fresh parsley, chopped

DIRECTIONS

Place the olive oil in a pan and saute' with garlic and onion; cook for approximately 30 seconds to one minute. If you are using canned tomatoes, crush or chop finely. For fresh tomatoes, chop them up in small cubes. Add white wine and saute' for three to four minutes. Add basil, oregano, salt and pepper to taste. Serve over spaghetti or linguini and sprinkle with freshly chopped parsley.

LINGUINI WITH GARLIC, MUSHROOMS, AND PARSLEY

INGREDIENTS

2 tablespoons olive oil

6 garlic cloves

One 12 ounce carton mushrooms

1 large bunch of parsley

1 ounce white wine

Freshly ground pepper

Freshly grated Parmesan cheese

DIRECTIONS

Into a frying pan place the olive oil and finely chopped garlic. Gently saute' for a couple of minutes. Add finely chopped mushrooms and chopped parsley. You may wish to use a food processor if available. Simmer. Add one ounce white wine. Serve over a bed of white linguini or fettuccine. Sprinkle with fresh parsley and add grated Parmesan cheese. Use freshly ground pepper to taste.

PASTA A LA SINATRA

INGREDIENTS

2 tablespoons olive oil

4 chopped garlic cloves

3 small onions

One 8 ounce jar sun-dried tomatoes

2 medium summer squash, finely chopped

Basil and fresh ground pepper to taste

Fettucine (¼ pound per person)

Grated parmesean cheese

Chopped parsley

DIRECTIONS

Place two tablespoons of olive oil in a saucepan. Add four chopped cloves of garlic and three small onions chopped up in fine pieces. Saute' the garlic and olive oil in the pan for a few minutes.

Put a jar of sun-dried tomatoes mixed with olive oil in the blender or food processor and process to desired consistency. Place this in the saucepan over the onions and garlic. Take two to three mid-sized summer squash and chop them in fine pieces. Place that into the frying pan and saute' over a low heat. Add fresh basil and pepper. Place this sauce over a bed of fettucini. Add grated cheese and garnish with chopped parsley.

SPINACH FETTUCCINE WITH A FRESH, MILD TOMATO SAUCE

INGREDIENTS

2 tablespoons olive oil

1 clove garlic, chopped

2 medium onions

6 medium tomatoes

Fresh basil, one small bunch, cut

Freshly grated Parmesan cheese

Freshly ground pepper

¼ pound pasta per person

DIRECTIONS

Place olive oil, finely chopped garlic, and onions in a frying pan and gently saute'. To remove the skin from tomatoes, place the tomatoes in a pot, cover with water and bring to gentle boil. After the water has boiled, take tomatoes out and peel skins which should remove easily. Don't overboil. Slice tomatoes up into fine pieces and add to the mixture of garlic, onion, and olive oil. Saute' in a frying pan for a few minutes. Add freshly cut strips of basil. Cook the pasta in a pot for two to three minutes and drain. Place fresh basil-tomato sauce on top. Sprinkle with grated cheese and fresh ground pepper to taste. This is a dry pasta dish, yielding little extra sauce.

PASTA SHELLS WITH ORGANIC SPINACH

INGREDIENTS

2 tablespoons olive oil

3 cloves garlic, diced

1 dozen mushrooms, finely sliced

2 bunches organically grown spinach

1 pound pasta shells

2 tablespoons Parmesan cheese

Fresh ground pepper

DIRECTIONS

Into large frying pan put 2 tablespoons olive oil. Add diced garlic or substitute one tablespoon dried flaked garlic and sliced mushrooms. Saute' over medium heat for a couple of minutes. Add two bunches of spinach. Cover frying pan and steam spinach for two minutes. Toss before serving. Spoon over pasta, one-quarter pound servings per person. Garnish with grated Parmesan cheese and add freshly ground pepper to taste.

PASTA WITH FENNEL AND TUNA

INGREDIENTS

1 pound fresh fennel

2 tablespoons olive oil

1 large onion

½ cup tomato sauce

½ tablespoon pine nuts

3 tablespoons dried black currants

Seasalt and fresh ground pepper

1 pound fresh tuna cut in one inch pieces

1 pound pasta (chef's choice)

6 threads saffron

Fresh parsley, chopped

DIRECTIONS

Boil the fennel until tender; drain and chop. Saute' the tuna and onion in olive oil and brown. Add tomato sauce and simmer. Add fennel, pine nuts, currants, seasalt and pepper to taste. Cook over a low heat. Add tuna and continue to simmer for approximately 20 minutes.

Prepare pasta according to package directions. Dissolve saffron into two tablespoons of warm water. Add saffron to dried cooked pasta and mix thoroughly. Spoon tuna sauce over pasta and serve with freshly chopped parsley as desired.

Rice with Steamed and Stir Fried Vegetables

Ingredients

2-3 ounces of water

2-3 medium sliced carrots

2 medium zucchini, chopped

1 small bunch of broccoli, chopped

2 medium summer squash, chopped

1 dozen mushrooms, chopped

¼ head of cauliflower, chopped

1 tablespoon dried garlic or 3 cloves fresh garlic (minced)

2 teaspoons dried basil

2 tablespoons olive oil

2 tablespoons Parmesean cheese

1 ½ cups short-grain brown rice (see brown rice recipe)

Fresh chopped parsley

Directions

Place into a wok or frying pan two to three ounces of water. Use a steaming rack if available. Place the chopped vegetables into the wok or frying pan and cover. Sprinkle garlic and crushed dried basil on top. Stir frequently if not using a rack. Heat and steam for several minutes until the vegetables are tender. When tender, sprinkle two tablespoons olive oil over the mixture and add fresh ground pepper to taste. Sprinkle freshly grated Parmesean cheese and freshly chopped parsley over the steamed vegetables and serve with short-grain brown rice.

FRIED RICE

INGREDIENTS

1 tablespoon dark sesame oil

1 medium onion, sliced

1 dozen mushrooms, sliced

½ package frozen peas

1 tablespoon shredded daikon

4 cups cooked short-grain brown rice

½ tablespoon tamari soy sauce

Chopped scallions or fresh chopped parsley

DIRECTIONS

Brush skillet with sesame oil. Heat for a minute or less but do not let oil start to smoke. Add onion, mushrooms, peas, and daikon; place rice on top. If rice is dry, moisten with a few drops of water. Cover skillet and cook on low heat for 10 to 15 minutes. Add tamari soy sauce and cook for another five minutes. Stir to mix before serving.

Garnish with scallions or chopped parsley.

BUCKWHEAT PANCAKES WITH BLUEBERRIES

INGREDIENTS

1 cup buckwheat flour

1 cup other whole grain flour

1 teaspoon baking powder

2 cups soymilk or water

2 egg whites

1 tablespoon canola oil

1 tablespoon honey

½ cup fresh unsweetened blueberries

DIRECTIONS

Stir dry ingredients together. Add soymilk, egg whites, oil and honey and mix briefly. Add blueberries and stir gently. Cook on hot, lightly oiled griddle.

This is my version of a recipe taken from *Fighting Radiation with Foods, Herbs, and Vitamins*—Documented Natural Remedies that Boost Your Immunity and Detoxify, (Vitality, Inc., 1990), by Steven R. Schechter.

Chicken with Peapods and Zucchini

Ingredients

Boneless breast of chicken

2 tablespoons peanut or olive oil

12 sliced mushrooms

1 teaspoon dried basil, crushed

2 cloves garlic, crushed, or one tablespoon dried garlic

1 tablespoon dried onion

1 medium zucchini, chopped

1 cup peapods

1 ounce white wine

Grated Parmesan cheese

Brown rice (see brown rice recipe)

Fresh parsley, chopped

Directions

Slice boneless breast of chicken into two inch by ½ inch strips. Heat two tablespoons of peanut or olive oil in wok or fry pan. Add chicken, mushrooms, dried basil, garlic, onion, zucchini, peapods. Spoon-saute' until chicken is done. Add peapods and one ounce of white wine (optional). Simmer gently until zucchini and peapods are tender. Serve over pasta with grated cheese, or serve with brown rice. Garnish with parsley.

CHICKEN WITH ARTICHOKES

INGREDIENTS

Boneless breast of chicken

2 tablespoons peanut or olive oil

1 teaspoon crushed dried basil

2 cloves garlic or one tablespoon dried garlic

12 thinly sliced mushrooms

1 ounce white wine

1 large or two small jar(s) marinated artichoke hearts (drained)

½ lemon

Fresh parsley, chopped

DIRECTIONS

Slice boneless breast of chicken in two inch by ½ inch strips. Heat two tablespoons peanut or olive oil in wok or fry pan. Add chicken, one teaspoon crushed dried basil and two cloves garlic or dried garlic. Spoon-saute'. Add one dozen thinly sliced mushrooms, one ounce white wine (optional) and one large or two small jar(s) artichokes. Squeeze ½ lemon on top and mix. Garnish with fresh parsley and serve.

VARIATION

ADDITIONAL INGREDIENTS

Bread crumbs

Fresh ground pepper

DIRECTIONS

Slice chicken into larger pieces, four inch by two inch strips. Sprinkle with olive oil, chopped parsley, chopped garlic, bread crumbs, and with pepper. Grill ninety seconds on charcoal grill or until bread crumbs are brown. Place in bowl and squeeze lemon juice over it; add artichokes and serve.

SANTIAGO'S CHICKEN

INGREDIENTS

4 boneless breasts of chicken

4 cloves of garlic, chopped

½ cup dry sherry or white wine

1 fresh lime

1 teaspoon paprika

½ teaspoon coriander

½ teaspoon cumin

½ teaspoon ginger

Seasalt and freshly ground pepper to taste

Fresh parsley, chopped

DIRECTIONS

Place the boneless breasts of chicken in a dish and add remaining ingredients, excluding parsley, to form a marinade. Place in refrigerator for at least one to two hours. Turn the chicken every so often to coat evenly with marinade.

Cook over a charcoal or mesquite fire; grill chicken until it is tender, continuing to baste with marinade while cooking. Garnish with freshly chopped parsley.

BREADED SOLE, FLOUNDER OR FLUKE

INGREDIENTS

2 tablespoons olive oil

1 ounce white wine

Fish fillets

Italian style breadcrumbs

1 lemon

½ teaspoon basil

Seasalt and freshly ground pepper

Watercress

Fresh parsley, chopped

DIRECTIONS

Prepare marinade using the olive oil, wine, the juice of one lemon, basil, and parsley, seasalt and pepper to taste. Dip fish in this marinade and then gently role it in bread crumbs. Grill the fish over a hot charcoal fire for only a minute or two on each side. Serve with lemon slices and garnish with chopped parsley and/or watercress.

GRILLED TUNA OR SWORDFISH WITH SPINACH

INDREDIENTS

1 tablespoon olive oil

1 bunch of spinach

1 fresh lemon

1 pound fresh tuna or swordfish

1 teaspoon basil

Seasalt and fresh ground pepper

Fresh parsley, chopped

DIRECTIONS

Into a sauce pan, add one tablespoon of olive oil. Rinse the spinach, discharging the stems, and place it wet into the frying pan and cover. Simmer for a few minutes but do not overcook. Squeeze lemon over fish and sprinkle with seasalt, pepper, and basil crushed between the palms of your hands. On a hot charcoal grill, place the tuna and cook only two to three minutes per side. Tuna should be slightly red in the middle. Remember that tuna does not need to be uniform throughout in its color. Rare tuna, like rare meat, tastes very good. If you grill a swordfish you will need to grill longer, at least until there is uniform color throughout the meat. After the fish is cooked, take the spinach out of the pan and place on a platter. Place the fish on top of the spinach, squeeze some fresh lemon over it. Sprinkle with fresh parsley and serve.

MARINATED BLUEFISH

INGREDIENTS

2 medium sized bluefish steaks

½ lemon

2 tablespoons olive oil

1 ounce white wine

½ teaspoon crushed dried basil

3 cloves garlic, finely chopped

Seasalt and fresh ground pepper

Fresh parsley, chopped

DIRECTIONS

Place bluefish steaks on a platter and squeeze fresh lemon on top. Mix olive oil, white wine, basil, garlic and pepper and pour over fish. Marinate for several hours or overnight if desired. Saute' in a lightly oiled frying pan or grill on an open fire. Add marinade to the saute'. Sprinkle with fresh parsley and serve. This dish is served nicely over rice, accompanied by a watercress salad.

EYE OF ROUND ROAST WITH ROSEMARY AND POTATOES

INGREDIENTS

2 pound eye of the round roast

Rosemary, crushed in a small bowl

Seasalt

Freshly ground pepper

8 small red potatoes cut in half

2 onions, sliced

2 tomatoes, sliced

Fresh parsley, chopped

DIRECTIONS

Trim off excess fat from the roast and sprinkle with crushed rosemary, seasalt, and freshly ground pepper to taste. Place the roast on a rack in roasting pan and add one ounce of water. Place potatoes around roast and sprinkle with rosemary. Reheat oven to 350 degrees and then roast till tender, approximately one and a half hours. Slice thin and serve with raw sliced onions and tomatoes, sprinkled with fresh parsley.

LOW-FAT EXCEPTIONAL HAMBURGERS

INGREDIENTS

2 pounds top round steak or London broil, ground

Few drops extra virgin olive oil

Seasalt and freshly ground pepper

Fresh parsley, chopped

DIRECTIONS

Ask the butcher to weigh the meat and then trim off all the fat. Grind the round steak or roast. Knead the meat into quarter-pound hamburgers.

Into a cast iron or steel frying pan, add a few drops of extra virgin olive oil and place the hamburgers over a high heat. Sprinkle with seasalt and fresh ground pepper to taste. When cooked serve with freshly chopped parsley.

This is the most nutritious way to have meat. Each quarter pound of the steak includes only four to five grams of fat per serving. This is an excellent recipe for those who desire red meat.

FOODS TO AVOID

Lard, most margarines, coconut oil, palm oil, salt pork, suet, bacon, meat drippings, gravies, cream sauces, catsup, mayonnaise, and most especially butter.

Whole milk, cream, sour cream, non-dairy coffee creamer, whipped toppings, and particularly cheese.

Red meat, fatty meats, spareribs, pork, ham, corned beef, regular ground meat, cold cuts, hot dogs, sausages, bacon, meats canned or frozen in sauces or gravies, frozen packaged dinners, fried fish, fried meats, egg yolk, duck, poultry skin, shrimp, sardines, fish roe, and most importantly organ meats and peanut butter.

White flour and commercial products utilizing it including biscuits, muffins, sweet rolls, doughnuts, waffles and french toast. Also to be avoided are french fries, potato chips, junk foods, popcorn with salt or butter.

Olives, creamed or fried vegetables, and avocado.

Cream soups, dehydrated soups, and commercial bouillon.

All beverages with added sweeteners, alcohol, and caffeine.

(coffee, one cup/day)

Pies, cakes, cookies, chocolate, coconut, cashew and macadamia nuts, candies, jams, jellies, maple syrup, sugar, molasses, and expecially ice cream.

FOODS TO SUBSTITUTE

Cold-pressed extra virgin olive oil, canola oil, flax linseed oil, safflower oil, corn oil, unsaturated margarines in small amounts, and meat juices.

One percent milk, low fat cottage cheese, skim milk cheese, riccota cheese.

Fresh fish two to three times per week, lean beef one to two times per week only, egg whites, one whole egg (250 mg cholesterol) per week, lean veal and lamb, lobster, scallops, crab in small amounts, chicken, turkey, wild goose, tuna fish (water packed), dried beans, lentils, pasta, rice, potatoes, barley, buckwheat, millet, peas, seaweed, and tofu.

Graham crackers, whole-wheat and rye bread, pita bread, baked goods containing no whole milk, egg yolk or sugar, unsweetened cereals, unsalted and unbuttered popcorn.

Celery, cauliflower, zucchini, daikon (white radish), green beans, broccoli, squash, kale, onions, garlic, cabbage, parsley, mushrooms, watercress, spinach.

Chicken soup (no fat), clear broth, fat-free vegetable soup, and most importantly, MISO soup.

Fresh squeezed juice, or unsweetened frozen or canned juice, mineral water, herbal teas.

Angelfood cake, puddings made with skim milk, frozen yogurt, cooked apples, all fresh fruit, unsweetened frozen or canned fruit (drained), rice pudding, chestnuts, and almonds.

CHAPTER 13

WHO IS THIS NEW PERSON IN THE MIRROR

This chapter will deal with the many repercussions, both positive and negative, of weight loss. The text will support you in handling the multitude of new challenges you will now face, including keeping the weight off.

Since any change often brings up deep emotions and feelings, losing a great deal of weight may create some unforeseen problems. As these feelings and situations come up, it will be tempting for you to go back to your previous maladaptive yet familiar ways of handling them. Remember, we often use food as a substitute when we are hungry for something else. We eat when we are alone, sad, depressed, frustrated, or even happy for that matter, as we often turn to food unconsciously. The toxic effects of repressed anger can also drive us to eat voraciously, yet without awareness.

As I mentioned before, it is the unconscious drives that really motivate us and at times control us. This is the reason why outside feedback and support is so helpful in learning about ourselves. There are similar threads of experience that overweight people face and share. In emotional support groups, we can experience the sharing and caring of others who have the same pain and conscious struggles over obesity. While we may not be aware of our own unconscious issues, group support can sometimes bring them out as we relate and react to others' issues that we may then realize are ours as well. Through them we can see ourselves. Mood swings, for example, are common after losing a considerable amount of weight. You may feel elated, proud of yourself, excited about your future, or *sexy*, as well as sad, scared, defensive, and lost. These feelings will modify in time, but in the meantime, it helps to have someone who understands what you are going through to encourage and support you.

Not only will *You* have a reaction to your new self, but people you have known for years who are accustomed to you as a fat person are going to have various reactions to the new you, ranging from total support and an expression of being happy to becoming jealous of you, judging you, possibly rejecting you, or perhaps even coming on sexually to you. *Get ready!* If you are oversensitive to others' opinions of you, their forces can be counterproductive to all your hard work. No one is able to be consistent all the time. We all have our ups and downs. You might have a friend who validates you often. If you begin to rely on her for a sense of yourself, what happens when she is having a terrible day, or week, or even year? What happens when she is feeling particularly insecure or angry? She can inadvertently pull that validation away, and if you are dependent on her for validation, you may start feeling negated and worthless.

When you stop basing your value on having or not having a particular attribute, you will feel 100 percent better about everything. *You must begin to realize that your self-worth is not about anything you do.* You are worthy simply because you exist. It is wonderful to grow and heal and change for the better, but it is not as if you will be more worthy when you do it. This kind of *conditional acceptance* sets up relentless expectations of what you *have* to change in order to be loved, lovable, happy, or worthy. Unfortunately, our society programs us to believe in this destructive setup. Thus, the man who is incredibly sensitive, creative, loving, hardworking, and earning a moderate yet respectable living can be seen as less valuable than the millionaire CEO of a major corporation who may have little integrity and be ruthless and uncaring, destroying the morale of his personnel, or the environment for that matter. This is a trap. *Only you can change yourself* – your beliefs and perceptions. It will take a longer time period for society to change its faulty belief system.

Having a stronger sense of self, of who you are and what's great about you, without validation from the outside is important to all people, fat and thin. While support groups can help you establish these beliefs about yourself, you have to take over the helm at some point. It is particularly crucial for you to be self-directed if you are going to keep the weight off because old foes and friends alike may tempt you to go back to the way you were, to the person they "knew or loved," that is, someone with whom they felt comfortable and unthreatened. *You can't stay stuck for anyone.* You may indeed become threatening, but this may be a gift to others. You might elicit feelings that cause them to look at themselves and their behavior just as you have. You may have a close friend who is still overweight express happiness for you, and yet you feel the opposite energy coming toward you from "underneath," which usually are his unconscious or subconscious feelings. He or she may not mean to be rejecting or cruel, but when people get frightened or jealous, triggering their own emotions on a deep level, they can act out on you and/or attack you in one way or another.

Any strong negative reaction is an indication that *they* very much want to change for the better too but feel stuck, or believe they can't, or are terrified to do so. Don't fall into the trap of then feeling guilty for your own good fortune. You've worked hard for this new body. You deserve it. You are not a bad person if they experience pain due to your healthier self. Stop feeling that it is your job to protect people from their pain. There is potential for change, growth and healing through this pain. Let others grow.

WEIGHT LOSS IS GREAT – CHANGE IS HARD

There are going to be many other changes and shifts that accompany your weight loss. You might be asking yourself the following questions:

Should I go out and buy a different wardrobe?

Do I have enough money to buy the clothes I need?

What if I gain the weight back after I buy all these clothes?

Should I change my image?

With my new image, should I change my hairstyle?

With my dress size diminishing, do I look too sexy?

Many of these questions will come up and many decisions will need to be made. My advice here is to *take your time.* When you are clear, the changes will come automatically. The new you is becoming more integrated and developing a deeper sense of self, meaning that you can trust your instincts to know what you want. With new awareness, you will start to get a new sense of what to do. Although you may change your look two or three times before you find the one that feels right, take the struggle out and enjoy this project.

You may begin to feel more sexual energy. With the loss of weight, your body may look more appealing. This may cause you to feel more alive and happy, or perhaps even guilty and frightened. But sexuality is a healthy part of life, and once viewed as such can bring much pleasure and satisfaction. If you feel a new sexual energy being directed at you, use it as a tool. If it frightens you, you may want to explore it with a professional counselor. If, on the other hand, it excites you, move with it. Flirt, play, have fun. Do not try to suppress these feelings for fear that something uncontrollable will happen to you. Your body is awakening and moving toward its natural urges. Accept it and allow it to happen.

Realize, though, that a husband or wife may go into fear of losing you because you are looking so terrific. Do your best to express your love and commitment to him or her. Accentuate the positive effects your transformation has on your spouse as well as you. Go out dancing. Create more romance. This could be an opportunity to ignite a delightful fire into your marriage. If, on the other hand, you are in an unfulfilling relationship, this may be the time to explore it. While I don't recommend taking on too many emotional issues at one time, neither do I suggest remaining stuck in a bad relationship. It is often difficult to let go of relationships, even destructive ones. It takes a certain conviction to heal your life, in wanting to surround yourself with people who are there for you most of the time, not trying to manipulate or control you, or use you to satisfy their needs at your expense. People hold on to destructive relationships for various reasons, sometimes out of fear of being alone. If you have connections that no longer work for you, that hurt you, then you owe it to yourself to see if you want to let them go or to work on them by restructuring the dynamics of the connection.

Be aware that in any recovery aspect, you need to take more responsibility for your actions and look at the negative patterns that you would like to change in your relationships as well as yourself. If you have a tendency to manipulate loved ones with your weight, the old pattern can show up if tensions are high at home. For example, if your spouse wanted you to lose weight and is now thrilled that you did, be careful not to reach for food if he or she upsets you. Remind yourself that you are the one who ultimately is punished by this action. Continue to find and utilize healthier ways to handle your strong emotions. If you are feeling angry and your old pattern was to eat, take note of the anger. Once you are in charge of it instead of it being in charge of you, you can channel it in a different direction. You can go out and *take a walk, go into the woods and scream, turn on some music and dance, walk the dog, go to a movie, or call a friend and share your feelings. Remember, patterns change with repetition of new behavior.* The more you take different action, the more you acknowledge your commitment to yourself. When you care enough to change, the new behavior will strengthen and so it becomes easier to follow.

Let's say you go home to visit your family. At dinner, your mother tries to serve you many items that your awareness knows are harmful. If, when you say, "No, thank you," you hear "But, I made this especially for you," you will know that you need to change your usual way of interacting with her. You may feel enraged. You may feel guilty and compelled to eat what you don't want to eat. But it is better to perhaps disappoint your mother than to betray yourself. If your mother expresses love through pushing food, and saying no indicates in her mind that you don't love her, you might try expressing that you appreciate the time she took to cook for you and that you love her, but that you have worked so very hard to change your eating habits that you must honor your commitments.

BE A FRIEND TO YOU!

This brings to mind the case of Sally, a school teacher who was in the weight-loss program I supervised. Sally weighed about 225 pounds when she started. At five feet three inches, she was round to say the least. Over the course of the program, she lost 70 pounds and really felt great about herself. In the two years since the program ended, Sally has kept off at least 50 pounds of the original weight, fluctuating within a

10-15 pound range. I spoke with her recently, and she is still determined to lose more. Her twin sister, on the other hand, was also in the program and while losing weight then, has put all of it back on. Now the relationship between the sisters is strained. Sally sometimes feels responsible for the tension, for having succeeded where her sister didn't, yet she knows she must honor herself and not go back to the old way of punishing herself. After she lost the weight, Sally wrote me and I share with you a portion of that letter:

"Smile 'tho your heart is aching," a corny song I suppose, and the rest of it just gets worse. What happens if you actually lived that line all your life?

I was taught how to love everyone, it helps build self-confidence and self-esteem in others, but wait, what about me? These characteristics are now growing within me with the weight-loss. I now have more energy to do more for others -- WRONG! That's the energy I need to turn inward toward myself. That's part of becoming the WHOLE me, not just the me who's becoming thinner. I have to do this for me, the person who needs to learn to relax and do things just for me. If I take the time to love and nurture myself, people will love me and I will love me, even though I have faults. People won't love me because I'm the person who can do it all . . .

. . . I'm not only going to have strong roots and growth, I'm going to BLOOM!

God didn't and won't sponsor any junk."

Love, as we can see, has incredible healing powers. Filling yourself up with food or even someone else's love will not fill the emptiness. But loving yourself will. And if you have a setback or become upset with yourself, and go through some turmoil that results in overeating, be careful not to turn your self-love into self-hate. If this does occur, catch it as soon as possible and *apologize for turning against yourself.* This may sound silly, but it works. Self-hate, or anger turned within, will only cause you to feel even more turmoil and possibly prolong or create another binge. If you slip up, remember to forgive yourself. Understand that it takes time to change these old patterns completely, and don't become greedy. If you have lost 25 pounds or have toned your stomach, but your legs still need work, look in the mirror with approval. Don't knock those legs. They need you now to love them as they are. In all the therapy I've done with women, their biggest issue was the size and shape of their legs. Perhaps this is because women feel that men place too much emphasis on legs. However, in the Men's Self-Awareness Group that I run, I've learned this is not the case.

FRIENDS OR FOOD POLICE?

Weight reduction is recovery and self-healing. Perfection is not the key to happiness. Be patient, but keep the momentum going. Take a few moments here and there to praise yourself and express gratitude. Look in the mirror and thank yourself out loud. This may also sound silly, but your mind needs this type of reinforcement, and speaking to yourself while looking into your own eyes is a powerful exercise. While others may support you or even unconsciously try to undermine you, you are the one who is ultimately responsible for your own feelings, your growth, your behavior, your happiness, and your body.

Friends may think they are being encouraging by being "food policemen," suggesting what you eat or don't eat. You can choose to respond to each situation accordingly. If they do indeed care, you can thank them for their suggestions, knowing in your heart that you are "recovering." On the other hand, a friend may think that something you are eating is bad for you while you know that in your program of awareness, you can balance the food with other less caloric items. You are responsible for your own choices. Only you know what truly is best for you. And if you are doing something that is not in your best interest, you will know it, and a gentle reminder may be all that you need to put you back on track. You are writing your own program and can create it according to your own taste and preferences. Support from friends is fine. Intrusion is not. While you may want an occasional reality check, simply be aware that others' reality may not be your own. And you must stay firmly within your own boundaries.

Checking your real feelings is a good way of staying in touch with yourself. When someone makes a comment that you know is true about yourself, you feel it in your gut. When they try to force their reality on you, however, you will feel an assault to your being and can tell them so. This is self-actualization and it requires a vigilance that many people would rather not face. These are exactly the confrontations that some people back away from by padding themselves with fat or acquiescing to everyone else's wants and needs. While this may or may not have been your old behavior, it certainly isn't part of the self-worth *Lose to Win* program.

Other friends may be consciously or unconsciously jealous of you, trying to undermine you. Friends, co-workers, and family members close to you who do not respond well at first to your transformation are resisting change. They were comfortable with you the way you were, so they may be reacting to losing the familiar. In due time, they will come back around and accept you. As a matter of fact, you may be feeling a loss yourself. If you have been overweight for many, many years, or have lost 60-100 pounds, it may feel as though you have lost a friend. Or if you have been using your weight to hide, you may feel a sense of fear in terms of how you will survive. This is where it is especially beneficial to look yourself in the eyes in the mirror and find comfort where you once may have seen rejection. In time, you will adjust and develop healthy ways to feel safe.

Again, taking quiet time to acknowledge that you love yourself is one such way to do this. Rejoicing in your weight loss is another. You may reward yourself by buying clothes in the regular-size department instead of the "big-is-beautiful" department. If you have been leading a reclusive life and begin to feel more alive and want to go out more often, do so. Or, like Roger Buffaloe, if you had trouble fitting into cars before, you may now physically and metaphorically love the pleasure of riding comfortably. As you participate in more activities that satisfy you and occupy your thoughts, you will be relieved of your preoccupation with your body. Allow yourself to enjoy your meals; put love into your food, especially when you prepare it for yourself and others. Food made with love tastes better. I know. My father taught me this, and his meals were always outstanding. I've never had a weight problem. I appreciate food and the love that goes into it, but I know it is only a symbol for the love of the people behind it.

As you adopt a new lifestyle that supports you in making changes, losing weight, and keeping it off, you will have helped everyone around you. You will have more energy available to give to others because you first gave to yourself, and you will give authentically only when and what you are able. You may be an inspiration to those who are close to you, exuding a positive energy that says "I've changed for the better. You can too." Our society desperately needs role models who offer hope. We can look back on that old person in the mirror and see our growth reflected in the symbol of our new image—an image of integration and self-love. As cliche as it may sound, I genuinely feel, *we all need hope, faith, and love.*

CHAPTER 14

LOSE TO WIN

This book has been a collection of chapters that can enable us to actively participate in our health and nutrition as well as our awareness in life. Although attitudes and belief systems are important in the stabilization of our ideals, we need to understand that every one of us can be open to change. Being able to change our prejudices, our negative habits, and our lifelong self-defeating patterns opens us up to growth. It is truly growth that makes life rewarding and worth living.

The goal of this book is to help you integrate your body, mind, and spirit as a way of seeking your true aliveness and satisfaction in life. We are each responsible for our own health and happiness. While "Life" may strike us unexpected blows, we can do as much as possible to turn around bad situations and try to prevent them. Healthy eating, exercise, and emotional release can be considered as preventive medicine. These are habits that will be with us for rest of our lives once we begin the pattern, and they do not require self-sacrifice, merely awareness.

A low-fat/high-fiber diet is but the first step. Throughout the book, I have stressed that we cannot deprive ourselves of good tasting meals and foods that we like. I included several of my *personal* recipes that are created with a healthy heart and trim, fit body in mind. I recommended eliminating very few products completely from the diet, but rather simply using less and substituting low-fat versions of old comfort foods for those that no longer fit a healthy lifestyle.

One such product that I would suggest are *Buffaloe Cakes and Buffaloe Cookies*. I feel I can recommend them as highly as I do olive oil, garlic, and onions. One cake has two to three grams of fat and seven grams of fiber, which is the equivalent of seven bowls of cream of wheat, fourteen cups of iceberg lettuce, or six cups of leaf lettuce. While cream of wheat and lettuce have trace fat, a tuna salad sandwich made with mayonnaise has 17 grams of fat – as much as a corned beef sandwich – and a hamburger has 21! You can see why I recommend eating one cake as a substitute for breakfast, lunch, or perhaps even a dessert.

I eat one Buffaloe Cake with two glasses of spring water and a piece of fruit for lunch almost every day. I hardly have time to break from the office for a full meal, and I find that the cookie is as filling as a sandwich, with much fewer fats and calories and twice the fiber. A seemingly low-cal sandwich made with tuna and mayonnaise on commercial whole-wheat bread has about 400 calories and only three grams of fiber. With the cookie, I am getting double the fiber and half the calories, which vary from 180-200 depending on the flavor. And there are a variety of five flavors to chose from, so I can eat a different one almost every day. Since I started this routine over a year ago, I have lost ten pounds – and I am eating as healthily as before. Enough said. You now know my favorite foods and my personal and professional recommendations for a healthy diet. Much, if not everything, I have written in this book I have incorporated into my own life. For me, life has been a journey, and one that continues.

THE BEST OFFENSE IS A GOOD DEFENSE

Our lives are governed and influenced by our thoughts, beliefs, and lifestyle patterns that can be as equally damaging to the mind as to the body. My waiting room is full of clients who have both chronic and acute illnesses. With their lifestyles of bourgeois diets, maladaptive habits, and overweight tendencies, some have waited too long. They come into my office wanting to be cured, yet frequently take no responsibility for their own condition or attempting to change it. My clients want me to give them relief. But I am not a magician, nor do I have any powers that can induce healing. I can't make a new body with pharmacological agents. I can't replace a heart that is ravaged with disease with a new healthy one. It all has to come through our lifestyle patterns – the way we live in the world now. Granted, many people who now have heart disease were not taught how to take care of themselves. It's hard to believe, but *preventive medicine in this country is not a major aspect of medical training, instruction, or energy.* Much of my generation, for example, grew up on junk foods. As a medical student, I was never taught about junk foods, but fortunately this is changing somewhat.

I was delighted to see in the **Archives of Internal Medicine,** June 1991, an article recommending a national effort to educate the public on the benefits of nutritional healing. The panel of physicians urged the medical community as well as the government, media, educational systems, and food industry to collaborate in this effort. Their recommendations, highlighted in the following table (**Table 22**), affect each of us and all should do our parts in healing ourselves and our families.

TABLE 22

RECOMMENDATIONS OF THE NATIONAL EDUCATION CHOLESTEROL PROGRAM

RECOMMENDATION B.1. – The panel recommends that healthy Americans, both adults and children, select, prepare, and consume foods that contain lower amounts of SFAs, total fat, and cholesterol.

RECOMMENDATION E.1. – The panel recommends that health professionals advise patients and the public to adopt the recommended eating patterns.

RECOMMENDATION F.1. – The panel recommends that food producers, manufacturers, and distributors increase the availability of good-tasting foods that are lower in SFAs, total fat, and cholesterol.

RECOMMENDATION F.2 – The panel recommends that the food industry participate actively in helping the public attain desirable eating patterns through labeling and advertising activities.

RECOMMENDATION F.3. – The panel recommends that food vendors and other food distribution sites participate actively in the national effort.

RECOMMENDATION F.4. – The panel recommends that the food industry, including food and animal scientists, food technologists, and nutritionists, continue to develop and modify foods to help the public meet the recommended eating patterns.

RECOMMENDATION G.1 – The panel recommends that the mass media provide information on a lower SFA, lower total fat, and lower cholesterol eating pattern.

RECOMMENDATION H.1 – The panel recommends that government facilitate attainment of healthful eating patterns by modifying policies and approaches.

RECOMMENDATION I.1 – The panel recommends that all public and private educational systems become active partners by disseminating information about the role of eating patterns in CHD prevention.

We need to educate our children by example. *Radiation is something I am genuinely concerned about.* Manufactured toxins that rage the earth are slowly and insidiously infiltrating our bodies and our planet. The evils of nature are prevailing and we are not winning the war against disease. The environmental toxicities, the receding ozone layer of the atmosphere, the polluted water, the viral epidemic of AIDS, and other malignant, life-threatening viruses that prevail are something that every human being needs to be concerned about. It is true that our planet is on the verge of a biological armageddon. Although I ponder about these things, I have greater dread about what my children's children will face. However, I do have some hope for the future.

There is a new generation of people and a new generation of doctors who have taken responsibility for ourselves, the environment, and the planet, for that matter. The doctors who have made the recommendations for the National Education Cholesterol Program believe that not only health professionals should be concerned with making efforts to improve the state of public health, but also *other* professionals. They are calling upon government to coordinate nutrition statements and policies emphasizing low-fat and healthy eating; they are asking the media to report these findings and to explain nutritional terms and information; they are asking food manufacturers to research and develop tasty low-fat and high-fiber food products.

This text has been a collection of facts, thoughts, and scientific papers, and folklore explaining in simple terms how to follow a lifestyle awareness program, utilizing nutritional and dietary approaches with an emphasis on exercise and emotional healing as adjuncts to a healthy lifestyle. Roger Buffaloe was an ordinary man who overcame great adversity in his life. I, too, am an ordinary doctor. With your help, perhaps among all of us, we can make a difference in the current and future health of the population.

TABLE 23

THE AMERICAN HEART ASSOCIATION

DIETARY GUIDELINES

1. Dietary fat intake should be less than 30 percent of total calories (I prefer 20 percent).
2. Saturated fat (SFA) intake should be less than 10 percent of total calories.
3. Polyunsaturated fat (PUFA) should not exceed 10 percent of total daily calories.
4. Cholesterol intake should not exceed 300 mg per day.
5. Carbohydrate intake should represent 50 percent or more total calories with emphasis on complex carbohydrates (I prefer 65-70 percent complex carbohydrates).
6. Protein intake should constitute the remainder of the calories.
7. Sodium intake should be limited to less than three grams per day.
8. Alcohol consumption is not recommended, but if consumed, should not exceed one ounce a day of ethanol or eight ounces of wine or 24 ounces of regular beer.
9. Total calories should be consumed with the goal of achieving and maintaining a person's recommended body weight.
10. Consumption of a wide variety of foods is encouraged.

From My Heart to Yours

As a clinical cardiologist, I know the heart is where everything comes together. I think many peoples' lives would change if they really and truly put their hearts into their actions. *Unfortunately, the heart of many of us is broken.* We may be lonesome and need to be fed on many different levels. Some of us need to be touched. Some need to give and others to receive. We are all searching and would like to have solutions. We all want cures. But the best remedy, in my opinion, comes from within. It comes from deep within our core. It comes with awareness, insight, and a genuine feeling of knowing. Are you hungry? Are you hungrier for a healthier and more productive life? The possibilities for self-healing are endless. I, like many of the rest of you, have fantasies. My fantasy is to acquire a higher spiritual, emotional, and physical awareness. It is my hope that this text will stimulate your inner self to seek out your highest power in adopting a body you really wish to live in. We have no other choice. If you wear out this body, where are you going to live next?

APPENDIX

Following is an eating regimen that I have prepared for increased health and subsequent weight loss. As it is not a "diet," it may be repeated over and over or mixed with other foods recommended in this book. The astericks mark those recipes that I include in the *Recipes for Life* chapter, so called because these are foods I have eaten for years without significant weight-gain nor continual loss. This is a balanced program of merely eating with awareness.

BREAKFASTS

1 Buffaloe Cookie
   2 8-oz. glasses water
1 frozen waffle
   Spreadable fruit
½ grapefruit
   1 bran muffin
2 whole-grain pancakes*
   Pure maple syrup, blueberries

1 bowl oatmeal
   1 glass fruit juice
1 cup low-fat yogurt
   1 piece whole wheat toast
1 bowl whole grain cereal
   1 cup 1% milk
Rice cake with honey
   Banana

LUNCHES

Leaf lettuce, tomato salad
   Low-fat goat or cottage cheese
   (lemon and olive oil dressing)
Salad of greens, turkey,
   Feta cheese, raw carrots
Bowl of pasta and vegetables
   Served hot or cold
Salad of greens and cold veggies
   Cold new potatoes and/or beans
Tuna packed in water

1 cup soup
   ½ sandwich
   (tuna, hummus, turkey)
Buffaloe Cookie, Miso Soup*
   2 8-oz. glasses water
1 cup yogurt, fresh fruit
   Whole-grain toasted bagel
Spinach, raw or sauteed
   Tomatoes, mushrooms
   (olive oil and lemon)

DINNERS

Fish
   Steamed broccoli
   Baked potato
Santiago's Chicken*
   Basmati rice
   Green salad
Stir-fried vegetables
   Brown Rice
Soup
   Salad and bread

Pasta
   Salad of greens
   Dad's Tomatoes*
Fish
   Sauteed spinach
   Yellow and green zucchini
Pasta
   Salad
Chicken
   Salad

HEIGHT/WEIGHT TABLE

MEN

HEIGHT INCHES	SMALL FRAME	MEDIUM FRAME	LARGE FRAME
62	128-134	131-141	138-150
63	130-136	133-143	140-153
64	132-138	135-145	142-156
65	134-140	137-148	144-160
66	136-142	139-151	146-164
67	138-145	142-154	149-168
68	140-148	145-157	152-172
69	142-151	148-160	155-176
70	144-154	151-163	158-180
71	146-157	154-166	161-184
72	149-160	157-170	164-188
73	152-164	160-174	168-192
74	155-168	164-178	172-197
75	158-172	167-182	176-202
76	162-176	171-187	181-207

To determine your ideal weight, find your height in the left-hand column. Then move across the page to the body frame that best describes you. For the purpose of this table, your body frame is "small" if you can wrap your left thumb and middle finger around your right wrist and have these two digits overlap. If the thumb and finger barely touch, then you have a "medium" body frame. If they don't touch at all, you have a "large" build.

Courtesy of Metropolitan Life Insurance Company

HEIGHT/WEIGHT TABLE

WOMEN

HEIGHT INCHES	SMALL FRAME	MEDIUM FRAME	LARGE FRAME
58	102-111	109-121	118-131
59	103-113	111-123	120-134
60	104-115	113-126	122-137
61	106-118	115-129	125-140
62	108-121	118-132	128-143
63	111-124	121-135	131-147
64	114-127	124-138	134-151
65	117-130	127-141	137-155
66	120-133	130-144	140-159
67	123-136	133-147	143-163
68	126-139	136-150	146-167
69	129-142	139-153	149-170
70	132-145	142-156	152-173
71	135-148	145-159	155-176
72	138-151	148-162	158-179

To determine your ideal weight, find your height in the left-hand column. Then move across the page to the body frame that best describes you. For the purpose of this table, your body frame is "small" if you can wrap your left thumb and middle finger around your right wrist and have these two digits overlap. If the thumb and finger barely touch, then you have a "medium" body frame. If they don't touch at all, you have a "large" build.

Courtesy of Metropolitan Life Insurance Company

BEVERAGES

	SERVING SIZE	CALORIES	SODIUM
Club Soda	12 ounces	0	75 (mg)
Cola, regular	12 ounces	150	14
Gatorade	12 ounces	39	123
Ginger Ale	12 ounces	125	25
Root Beer	12 ounces	150	49
Beer, regular	12 ounces	145	19
Beer, light	12 ounces	100	10
Wine, dessert	3.5 ounces	70	10
Wine, red	3.5 ounces	75	6
Wine, white	3.5 ounces	70	5
Apple juice	4.0 ounces	58	3.5
Apricot nectar	4.0 ounces	70.5	4.5
Carrot juice	4.0 ounces	55	36
Cranberry	4.0 ounces	75	5
Pineapple juice	4.0 ounces	70	1
Prune juice	4.0 ounces	90	5.5
Tomato juice	4.0 ounces	21	438
V-8	4.0 ounces	25	378
Grapefruit juice	4.0 ounces	50	1
Grape juice	4.0 ounces	80	3.5
Orange juice	4.0 ounces	55	1

BEANS/NUTS/SEEDS

FOOD	SERVING SIZE	CAL.	FAT (G)	% CAL/FAT	CHOL.	FIBER
Soybeans (Tofu) (cooked)	1 cup	234	10	38%	0	
Soybean curd	1 piece	86	5	52%	0	
Peanuts, roasted	¼ cup	210	18	77%	0	
Peanut Butter	2 Tbsp	188	16	76%	0	
Almonds, roasted	¼ cup	246	23	84%	0	
Walnuts, black (shelled and chopped)	¼ cup	196	18	82%	0	
Chick-peas	½ cup	135	2	45%	0	6.2
Kidney Beans	½ cup	110	TR		0	5.8
Lentils	½ cup	115	TR		0	2
Pinto Beans	½ cup	115	TR		0	5.3
Split Peas	½ cup	115	TR		0	5.1
Pork and Beans in tomato sauce	1 cup	311	6.6	19%	6	
Lima Beans (frozen cooked)	1 cup	168	0.2	1%	0	
Lima Beans (canned)	1 cup	163	0.5	2%	0	
Green Beans (fresh, frozen)	1 cup	34	0.1	2%	0	
Green Beans (canned)	1 cup	32	0.3	8%	0	
White Beans, navy (cooked)	1 cup	212	1.1	4%	0	
Yellow Beans, wax (frozen)	1 cup	28	0.3	9%	0	
Yellow Beans (canned)	1 cup	32	0.4	11%	0	
Sunflower Seeds (hulled)	1 Tbsp	51	4.3	75%	0	
Water Chestnuts	4 nuts	20	0.1	4%	0	
Macadamia Nuts	1 ounce	196	20.3	93%	0	
Pecans (chopped or pieces)	1 Tbsp	51	5.2	91%	0	

CEREAL

FOOD	SERVING SIZE	CAL.	FAT (G)	% CAL/FAT	CHOL.	FIBER
Cereal						
All Bran	⅓ cup	70	1	13%	0	8.6
Bran (unprocessed)	1 ounce	91	.4		0	NA
Bran Buds	1 cup	144	1.8	11%	0	NA
Cheerios	1 ¼ cup	110	2	16%	0	1.6
Corn Flakes	1 ¼ cup	110	Trace		0	.4
Corn Grits	1 cup	125	.2		0	NA
Cream of Wheat	¾ cup	105	Trace		0	.6
40% Bran Flakes	¾ cup	95	1	.9%	0	6.0
Fruit Loops	1 cup	110	1	.9%	0	.3
Granola	⅓ cup	125	5	36%	0	NA
Grape Nuts	¼ cup	100	Trace		0	2.2
Oatmeal	¾ cup	108	2	17%	0	2.8
Product 19	¾ cup	110	Trace		0	1.2
Puffed Rice	1 cup	55	Trace		0	.2
Raisin Bran	¾ cup	90	1	1%	0	3.6
Rice Krispies	1 cup	110	Trace		0	Trace
Shredded Wheat	⅔ cup	100	Trace		0	3.3
Special K	⅓ cup	110	Trace		0	.4
Sugar Frosted Flakes	¾ cup	110	Trace		0	.2
Total	1 cup	100	1	.9%	0	2.5
Wheat Chex	⅓ cup	110	1	.8%	0	NA
Wheat Germ	1 Tbsp	23	.7	27%	0	NA
Wheaties	1 cup	100	1	.9%	0	2.6

CURED MEATS

FOOD	SERVING SIZE	CALORIES	(G.) FAT	% CAL/FAT	(MG.) CHOL.
Bacon	3 slices	110	9	73%	16
Bologna	1 ounce	90	8	80%	16
Corned Beef Brisket	3 ounces	215	16	66%	83
Frankfurter	1	145	13	80%	23
Ham	3 ounces	205	14	61%	52
Ham/lean only	3 ounces	135	5	33%	47
Liverwurst	1 slice	60	5	75%	45
Pork Sausage	1 link	50	4	72%	11
Salami/cooked	1 ounce	70	6	77%	18
Salami/hard	1 slice	42	3	64%	8

DAIRY

FOOD	SERVING SIZE	CALORIES	(G.) FAT	% CAL/FAT	(MG.) CHOL.
Cheeses					
Parmesan, grated	1 Tbsp	25	2	72%	3
Ricotta (part skim milk)	½ cup	170	10	53%	38
Ricotta (whole milk)	½ cup	215	16	67%	62
Swiss	1 ounce	105	8	68%	26
American	1 ounce	105	9	77%	27
American (spread)	1 tbls	47	3	57%	9
Brie	1 ounce	95	8	76%	28
Cheddar	1 ounce	115	9	70%	30
Cottage cheese (creamed)	½ cup	110	5	41%	16
Cream cheese	1 ounce	100	10	90%	31
Mozzarella (part skim milk)	1 ounce	80	5	56%	15
Mozzarella (whole milk)	1 ounce	80	6	68%	22
Blue cheese	1 ounce	100	8.2	74%	21
Feta	1 ounce	75	6.0	72%	25

FOOD	SERVING SIZE	CALORIES	(G.) FAT	% CAL/FAT	(MG.) CHOL.
Cheeses (cont'd)					
Romano	1 ounce	110	7.6	62%	29
Velveeta	1 ounce	82	3.8	42%	16
Milk, creams, and milk products					
Milk, nonfat (dry)	¾ cup	81	.2		0
Milk, skim	1 cup	85	Trace		4
Milk, 1%	1 cup	102	2.6	23%	10
Milk, 2% fat	1 cup	120	5	37%	18
Milk, Whole	1 cup	150	8	48%	33
Milk, evaporated (canned, whole)	1 cup	338	19.1	51%	74
Milk, evaporated (canned, skim)	1 cup	200	.6	2.7%	10
Buttermilk	1 cup	100	2	18%	9
Chocolate milk	1 cup	210	8	34%	30
Cocoa mix w/water	1 cup	100	1	.9%	1
Condensed Milk (sweetened)	1 cup	980	27	25%	104
Cream, light (20.6% fat)	1 Tbsp	29	2.9	90%	10
Cream, whipping (light)	1 cup	699	73.9	95%	265
Cream, whipping (heavy)	1 cup	821	88.1	96%	326
Cream, half&half	1 Tbsp	20	2	90%	6
Cream, heavy	1 Tbsp	50	6	90%	21
Creamer (non-dairy)	1 Tbsp	33	2.1	57%	0
Sour cream	1 Tbsp	25	3	95%	5
Dessert Topping	1 tbls	33	2.1	69%	0
Yogurt, Low-fat (plain)	8 ounces	145	4	25%	14
Yogurt, Low-fat (with fruit)	8 ounces	230	2	7.8%	10
Yogurt (whole milk)	8 ounces	139	7.4	48%	29

FOOD	SERVING SIZE	CALORIES	(G.) FAT	% CAL/FAT	(MG.) CHOL.
Milk, creams, and milk products (cont'd)					
Yogurt, Frozen	8 ounces	244	3.0	11%	10
Milk Shake (Vanilla)	10 ounces	315	9	26%	33
Ice Cream (rich)	1 cup	349	23.7	61%	88
Ice Cream (reg)	1 cup	269	14.3	48%	59
Ice Cream (Eskimo Pie)	1	270	19.1	64%	35
Ice Cream (Sandwich 3 oz)	1	238	8.5	32%	34
Ice Milk (soft-serve)	1 cup	223	4.6	19%	13
Ice Milk (Hard)	1 cup	131	5.6	38%	18
Pudding mix (whole milk)	1 cup	322	7.8	22%	36
Pudding (instant) (whole milk)	1 cup	325	6.5	18%	36
Pudding mix (dry, low-cal)	4 ounces	100			
Eggs					
Egg, boiled	1 large	80	6	68%	274
Egg, fried	1 large	95	7	66%	278
Egg, scambled	1 large	110	8	65%	282
Egg white	1 large	15	Trace	-	0
Egg yolk	1 large	65	6	83%	272

DESSERTS

FOOD	SERVING SIZE	CALORIES	(G.) FAT	% CAL/FAT	(MG.) CHOL.
Cookies					
Brownie with Nuts and Frosting	1 small	100	4	36%	14
Butter Cookie	1 small	25	1	36%	NA
Chocolate Chip Cookie	1 medium	45	2	40%	1
Fig Bars	1 bar	55	1	16%	7
Gingersnap	3 small	50	1	16%	NA
Marshmallow with chocolate coating	1 cookie	55	2	38%	NA
Oatmeal Raisin	1 medium	60	2	30%	Trace
Sandwich Cookie	1 medium	50	2	36%	0
Sugar Cookie	1 medium	60	3	45%	7
Ice Creams (See Dairy)					
Pies (9" pie)					
Apple Pie	⅙ pie	405	18	40%	0
Banana Custard Pie	⅙ pie	335	14	38%	NA
Blueberry Pie	⅙ pie	380	17	40%	0
Cherry Pie	⅙ pie	410	18	39%	0
Lemon Meringue Pie	⅙ pie	355	14	35%	143
Mincemeat Pie	⅙ pie	430	18	38%	0
Pecan Pie	⅙ pie	575	32	50%	95
Pumpkin Pie	⅙ pie	320	17	48%	109
Puddings					
Butterscotch	½ cup	170	4	21%	17
Chocolate	½ cup	150	4	24%	15
Custard	½ cup	150	8	48%	139
Rice Pudding	½ cup	155	4	23%	15
Tapioca Pudding	½ cup	145	4	25%	15

FOOD	SERVING SIZE	CALORIES	(G.) FAT	% CAL/FAT	(MG.) CHOL.
Cakes					
Angel Food	½₂	125	Trace		0
Carrot with cream cheese icing	½₆	385	21	49%	74
Cheesecake, plain	½₂	280	18	58%	170
Chocolate w/icing	½₆	235	8	31%	37
Danish, plain	1 medium	220	12	49%	49
Doughnut, yeast	1 medium	235	13	50%	21
Poundcake	½₇ loaf	120	5	38%	32
Spice w/icing	½₆	270	8	26%	NA

FATS/VEGETABLE OILS

FOOD	SERVING SIZE	CALORIES	(G.) FAT	% CAL/FAT	(MG.) CHOL.
Butter	1 Tbsp	100	13	100%	31
Lard (animal shortening)	1 Tbsp	115	13	100%	12
Chicken Fat	1 Tbsp	126	14	100%	9
Margarine (imitation/diet)	1 Tbsp	50	5	90%	0
Margarine (regular/soft)	1 Tbsp	100	11	100%	0
Coconut Oil	1 Tbsp	120	14	100%	0
Corn Oil	1 Tbsp	125	14	100%	0
Cottonseed Oil	1 Tbsp	120	14	100%	0
Olive Oil	1 Tbsp	125	14	100%	0
Palm Kernel Oil	1 Tbsp	120	13.6	100%	0
Peanut Oil	1 Tbsp	125	14	100%	0
Soybean Oil	1 Tbsp	120	14	100%	0
Sunflower Oil	1 Tbsp	125	14	100%	0
Vegetable Shortening	1 Tbsp	115	13	100%	0

FISH/SHELLFISH

FOOD	SERVING SIZE	CALORIES	(G.) FAT	% CAL/FAT	(MG.) CHOL.
Bluefish	3 ounces	135	4	26%	59
Clams, raw	2 clams	25	1	36%	59
Cod	3 ounces	100	3	27%	50
Crab, softshell (fried)	1 medium	215	13	54%	87
Crab, steamed	3 ounces	80	2	22%	79
Crabmeat, canned	3 ounces	85	2	21%	84
Flounder	3 ounces	100	6	54%	50
Herring, pickled	3 ounces	190	13	61%	85
Lobster Tail, (steamed)	1 medium	100	1	9%	88
Mackerel	3 ounces	215	15	62%	94
Mussels, steamed	3 ounces	80	2	22%	42
Oysters, raw	3 ounces	55	1	16%	42
Salmon, canned	3 ounces	120	5	37%	34
Salmon	3 ounces	150	7	42%	36
Sardines, canned (in oil)	3 ounces	175	9	46%	85
Scallops, steamed	3 ounces	95	1	9%	45
Shrimp	7 medium	200	10	45%	168
Swordfish	3 ounces	150	7	42%	56
Trout	3 ounces	215	14	58%	55
Tuna, chunk in oil (drained)	3 ounces	169	7	37%	NA
Anchovies	5 fillets	135	2	13%	NA
Herring, Pacific	3 ounces	153	8	47%	NA
Catfish	1 ounce	29	1	31%	0
Halibut, broiled	1 ounce	28	.3	9%	14
Sole	1 ounce	26	.3	10%	0

FRUITS

FOOD	SERVING SIZE	CAL.	FAT (G)	%CAL/FAT	CHOL.	FIBER
Apple	1 medium	90	Trace	-	0	2.8
Applesauce	½ cup	95	Trace	-	0	2
Apricots	3 apricots	50	Trace	-	0	2.2
Avocado	1 medium	325	31	86%	0	4.5
Banana	1 medium	105	1	-	0	2.1
Blueberries	½ cup	40	Trace	-	0	2.5
Cantaloupe	½ medium	95	1	-	0	2.7
Cherries, Canned	½ cup	105	Trace	-	0	1.7
Coconut	1 cup	277	282	91%	0	NA
Cranberry Sauce (canned)	¼ cup	105	Trace	-	0	NA
Dates	10 dates	219	.4	-	0	NA
Figs, dried	1 fig	50	Trace	-	0	3.7
Fruit cocktail (canned, water)	1 cup	91	.2	-	0	NA
Grapefruit	½ medium	40	Trace	-	0	1.7
Grapes, seedless	10 grapes	35	Trace	-	0	.4
Honeydew cubes	1 cup	60	Trace	-	0	1.2
Lemon	1 medium	15	Trace		0	NA
Mango	1 medium	135	Trace	-	0	2.9
Nectarine	1 medium	65	1	-	0	1.9
Orange	1 medium	60	Trace	-	0	1.6
Peach	1 medium	35	Trace	-	0	1.4
Pear	1 medium	100	1	-	0	5
Pineapple	½ cup	40	Trace	-	0	1.2
Plum	1 medium	35	Trace	-	0	1.4
Prunes, dried	5 large	115	Trace	-	0	7.9
Raisins	½ cup	220	Trace	-	0	4.9
Raspberries, raw	1 cup	70	.6	-	0	NA
Rhubarb, frozen (sweetened)	1 cup	381	.3	-	0	NA
Strawberries	1 cup	55	.7	-	NA	
Tangerine	1 large	46	.2	-	0	NA
Watermelon (diced pieces)	1 cup	42	.3	-	0	NA

GRAIN PRODUCTS – BREADS, PASTA, RICE

FOOD	SERVING SIZE	CAL.	FAT (G)	% CAL/FAT	CHOL.	FIBER
Bagel	1 bagel	200	2	9%	0	NA
Corn Bread	1 piece	200	7	31%	0	1.7
Frank/Burger Bun	1	115	2	15%	Trace	NA
French Bread	1 slice	100	1	9%	0	1.3
French Toast	1 slice	155	7	40%	112	NA
Hard Roll	1	155	2	11%	Trace	NA
Pancake, plain	1	60	2	30%	16	NA
Rye Bread	1 slice	65	1	13%	0	.9
Taco Shell	1	50	2	36%	NA	NA
Tortilla, corn	1 cake	65	1	13%	NA	NA
White Bread	1 slice	65	1	13%	0	.5
Whole Wheat Bread	1 slice	70	1	12%	0	1.4
Graham Crackers	2	60	1	15%	0	2.8
Melba Toast	1	20	Trace		0	NA
Saltine Crackers	4	50	1	18%	5	.5
Blueberry Muffin	1	135	5	33%	19	NA
Bran Muffin	1	125	6	43%	24	NA
Corn Muffin	1	145	5	31%	23	NA
English Muffin	1	140	1	6%	0	NA
Egg Noodles	1 cup	200	2	9%	50	1.7
Macaroni	1 cup	190	1	4%	0	1.2
Spaghetti	1 cup	190	1	4%	0	1.6
Rice, brown	½ cup	115	1	7%	0	2.4
Rice, white	½ cup	110	Trace		0	.1

MISCELLANEOUS

FOOD	SERVING SIZE	CALORIES	(G.) FAT	% CAL/FAT	(MG.) CHOL.
Beef - vegetable stew	1 cup	220	11	45%	71
Chili with beans	1 cup	340	16	42%	28
Corned Beef Hash	1 cup	290	10	31%	NA
Macaroni and Cheese	1 cup	340	22	46%	44
Spaghetti, canned	1 cup	260	9	31%	8
Biscuit with sausage and egg	1	555	37	60%	259
Cheeseburger Patty	4 ounces	525	31	53%	104
Chicken Nuggets	6	265	16	54%	60
Chicken Sandwich	1	615	34	49%	68
Enchilada	1	235	16	61%	19
Fish Sandwich with cheese	1	420	23	49%	56
Frankfurter	1	280	16	51%	45
French Fries	1 serving	230	12	46%	NA
Ham and Cheese Sandwich	1	400	22	49%	60
Onion Rings	1 serving	260	15	51%	NA
Pizza with cheese	1 slice	290	9	27%	55
Roast Beef Sandwich	1	345	13	33%	55
Taco	1	195	11	50%	21
Bacon Bits	1 tsp	14	0.6	38%	0
M & M Candy	¼ cup	230	9.7	37%	3
Potato Chips	10 chips	114	7	63%	
Olives, green	10	33	4	99%	
Beef Tongue	1 slice	49	3.3	60%	18
Beef Liver	1 ounce	40	1.1	24%	86
Beef Tallow, suet	1 Tbsp	120	13.2	99%	11
Pork-Deviled Ham	¼ cup	198	18.2	82%	5
Sausage, Vienna (canned)	1 whole	56	5.2	3%	10

POULTRY

FOOD	SERVING SIZE	CALORIES	(G.) FAT	% CAL/FAT	(MG.) CHOL.
Chicken, dark meat (with skin)	4 ounces	286	17	54%	103
Chicken, dark meat (no skin)	4 ounces	233	11	41%	105
Chicken, lt meat (with skin)	4 ounces	253	12	42%	96
Chicken, lt meat (no skin)	4 ounces	193	5	24%	96
Chicken breast (no skin)	½ breast	140	3	19%	73
Chicken breast (no skin, fried)	½ breast	160	4	22%	78
Chicken drumstick (with skin)	one	110	6	49%	48
Chicken drumstick (no skin)	one	75	2	24%	41
Duck with skin	4 ounces	380	32	75%	101
Duck no skin	4 ounces	227	13	52%	95
Turkey, dark meat (with skin)	4 ounces	253	13	47%	101
Turkey, dark meat (no skin)	4 ounces	213	8	33%	96
Turkey, lt meat (with skin)	4 ounces	220	9	38%	86
Turkey, lt meat (no skin)	4 ounces	180	4	20%	79
Chicken gizzard	4 ounces	108	2.4	20%	142

RED MEAT

FOOD	SERVING SIZE	CALORIES	(G.) FAT	% CAL/FAT	(MG.) CHOL.
Beef chuck roast	4 oz.	413	32	69%	117
Beef flank steak	4 oz.	306	17	57%	80
Beef rib roast	4 oz.	433	36	74%	96
Beef top round*	4 oz.	210	5	21%	70
Beef shortribs	4 oz.	533	48	81%	107
Beef sirloin*	4 oz.	233	9	36%	101
Beef T-bone*	4 oz.	240	12	45%	91
Beef tenderloin	4 oz.	233	10	41%	96
Hamburger (lean)	4 oz.	326	21	58%	112
Porterhouse steak*	4 oz.	246	12	43%	90
Lamb leg	4 oz.	213	8	33%	80
Lamb loin chop*	1 large	250	14	50%	60
Lamb rib chop*	1 large	290	22.5	70%	75
Pork loin chop*	1 medium	275	19	62%	84
Pork tenderloin	4 oz.	186	5	25%	87
Spareribs	4 oz.	453	37	68%	137
Veal cutlet	4 oz.	207	5.3	23%	112
Veal loin chop	4 oz.	246	13	34%	116
Veal rib roast	4 oz.	344	24	63%	119

MOST PREFERRED

Top round
Pork tenderloin
Veal cutlet

*All visible fat removed before cooking

SOUP CANNED, CONDENSED

FOOD	SERVING SIZE	CALORIES	(G.) FAT	% CAL/FAT	(MG.) CHOL.
Bean w/bacon	1 cup	170	6	31%	3
Beef Consomme	1 cup	15	1	60%	Trace
Chicken Broth	1 cup	40	1	22%	1
Chicken Noodle	1 cup	75	2	24%	7
Chicken Rice	1 cup	60	2	30%	7
Clam Chowder (red)	1 cup	80	2	22%	2
Clam Chowder (white)	1 cup	165	7	38%	22
Minestrone	1 cup	85	3	31%	2
Mushrooms w/milk	1 cup	205	14	61%	20
Split Pea w/ham	1 cup	190	4	18%	8
Tomato	1 cup	85	2	21%	0
Vegetable/vegetarian	1 cup	70	2	25%	0
Vegetable w/beef	1 cup	80	2	22%	5
Cream of Celery with water	1 cup	86	5.5	57%	7
Cream of Chicken with water	1 cup	94	5.8	55%	8
Canned Onion w/water	1 cup	65	2.4	33%	6
Dehydrated Onion	1 pack	150	4.6	27%	0

VEGETABLES

FOOD	SERVING SIZE	CAL.	FAT (G)	%CAL/FAT	CHOL.	FIBER
Artichoke, bud or globe (frozen)	1 whole	52	0.2	3%	0	
Asparagus	6 spears	20	Trace	-	0	2.2
Beets	½ cup	25	Trace	-	0	2.2
Broccoli	1 spear	55	Trace	-	0	4.5
Brussels Sprouts	1 cup	51	0.3	5%	0	
Cabbage, cooked	½ cup	15	Trace	-	0	2
Cabbage, raw (shredded)	½ cup	10	Trace	-	0	0.7
Carrot, raw	1 medium	30	Trace	-	0	2.4
Carrot, sliced (cooked)	½ cup	35	Trace	-	0	2.3
Cauliflower	½ cup	15	Trace	-	0	1.6
Celery, raw	1 stalk	5	Trace	-	0	0.7
Corn	½ cup	90	1	1%	0	3.9
Corn, creamed	½ cup	210	2.8	12%	0	
Cucumber, raw	½ cup	5	Trace	-	0	0.5
Eggplant, cubes	1 cup	25	Trace	-	0	4
Greens, Collard	1 cup	51	0.7	12%	0	
Lettuce, Iceberg	1 cup	5	Trace	-	0	0.5
Lettuce, Leaf	1 cup	10	Trace	-	0	1.2
Mushrooms, raw (sliced)	½ cup	10	Trace	-	0	0.9
Okra, frozen (cooked)	1 cup	70	0.2	2%	0	
Onion, raw (chopped)	½ cup	25	Trace	-	0	2.6
Peas, Chinese	½ cup	35	Trace	-	0	1.3
Peas, Green	½ cup	65	Trace	-	0	4.1
Pepper, Green (raw)	1 medium	20	Trace	-	0	0.8
Pepper, Jalapeno (raw)	1	7	0	-	0	

FOOD	SERVING SIZE	CAL.	FAT (G)	% CAL/FAT	CHOL.	FIBER

Vegetables (cont'd)

FOOD	SERVING SIZE	CAL.	FAT (G)	% CAL/FAT	CHOL.	FIBER
Pepper, Jalapeno (canned)	1	5	0	-	0	
Pickles, Dill	1 large	15	0.3	18%	0	
Pickles, Sweet	2 slices	11	0	-	0	
Potato, baked (no skin)	1 medium	145	Trace	-	0	3.7
Potato, boiled	1 medium	115	Trace	-	0	2.7
Radishes	4 medium	5	Trace	-	0	0.5
Sauerkraut (canned)	½ cup	20	Trace	-	0	2.4
Spinach, frozen	½ cup	30	Trace	-	0	2.1
Squash, Summer	1 cup	25	0.2	7%	0	
Squash, Winter	½ cup	40	1	22%	0	3.6
Sweet Potato (mashed)	½ cup	170	Trace	-	0	3.8
Tomato, raw	1 medium	25	Trace	-	0	1
Tomato Juice	½ cup	20	Trace	-	0	NA
Tomato Puree	½ cup	50	Trace	-	0	NA
Turnip, green	1 cup	38	0.5	11%	0	
Yam, cubes	½ cup	80	Trace	-	0	2.6
Vegetable Juice Cocktail	½ cup	20	Trace	-	0	NA
Zucchini, sliced (cooked)	½ cup	15	Trace	-	0	2.7

SELECTED REFERENCES

BOOKS

American College of Sports Medicine. Guidelines for Exercise Testing and Prescription. Philadelphia: *Lea & Febiger, 1986.*

Bailey C. Fit or Fat? Boston: *Houghton Mifflin Co, 1978.*

Balch JF and Balch PA. Prescription for Nutritional Healing. Garden City Park, NY: *Avery Publishing Group Inc, 1990.*

Bass E, Davis C. The Courage to Heal. New York: *Harper & Row, 1988.*

Bland J. Medical Applications of Clinical Nutrition. New Canaan, CT: *Keats Publishing, 1983.*

Bliznakof EG, Hunt GL. The Miracle Nutrient Coenzyme Q_{10}. New York: *Bantam Books, 1986.*

Bruch H. Eating Disorders. New York: *Basic Books, 1973.*

Carper J. The Food Pharmacy. Dramatic New Evidence That Food Is Your Best Medicine. New York: *Bantam Books, 1988.*

Cowmeadow O. An Introduction to Macrobiotics – The Natural Way to Health and Happiness. Wellingborough, Northamptonstine, Eng: *Thorsons Publishers Limited, 1987.*

Eastwood MA, Brydon WG, Tadesse K. "Effects of fiber on colon continence." Medical Aspects of Dietary Fiber. Spiller GA, McP Kay R, eds. New York and London: *Plenum Medical Books, 1980.*

Eliot RS, Breo DL. Is It Worth Dying For? New York: *Bantam Books, 1986.*

Fletcher AM. "How to Put More Fish and Omega-3 Fish Oils into Your Diet for a Longer, Healthier Life." Eat Fish, Live Better. New York: *Harper and Row, 1989.*

Goodwin J, et al. Sexual Abuse. Chicago: *Year Book Medical Publishers, 1989.*

Hirschmann JR, Munter CH. Overcoming Overeating. New York: *Fawcett Columbine, 1988.*

Hirschmann JR, Zaphiropoulos L. Are You Hungry. New York: *Random House, 1985.*

Hubert E, Soben A. "Properties and fatty acid composition of fats and oils." Handbook of Biochemistry. pp E-20-21. Cleveland: *CRC Press, 1970.*

JARVIS DC. Folk Medicine. New York: *Fawcett Crest, 1958.*

JENSEN B. Food Healing for Man. Escondido, CA: *Bernard Jensen Publisher, 1983.*

JOHNSTON IM AND JOHNSTON JR. PASSWATER RS, ED. AND MINDELL E. Flaxseed (Linseed) Oil and the Power of Omega-3. How to Make Nature's Cholesterol Fighters Work for You. New Canaan, CT: *Keats Publishing Inc, 1990.*

KUSHI M WITH JACK A. Diet for a Strong Heart. New York: *St. Martin's Press, 1985.*

LESSER M. Nutrition and Vitamin Therapy. New York: *Grove Press Inc, 1980.*

MASQUELIER J. "The bactericidal action of certain phenolics of grapes and wine." The Pharmacology of Plant Phenolics. New York: *Academic Press;1959.*

MEISELMAN K. Incest. San Francisco: *Jossey-Bass, 1986.*

MILLER A. For Your Own Good. New York: *Farrar, Straus, Giroux, 1983.*

MILLER A. Prisoners of Childhood. New York: *Basic Books, 1981.*

NATIONAL ACADEMY OF SCIENCES. Diet and Health: Implications for Reducing Chronic Disease Risk. Washington: *National Academy Press, 1989.*

NIAZI SK. The Omega Connection. The Facts About Fish Oils and Human Health. Chicago: *Esquire Books Inc, 1987.*

ORNISH D. Dr. Dean Ornish's Program for Reversing Heart Disease. The Only System Scientifically Proven to Reverse Heart Disease Without Drugs or Surgery. New York: *Random House, 1990.*

PEARSON D, SHAW S. Life Extension, a Practical Scientific Approach. New York: *Warner Books, 1982.*

PENNINGTON JAT. Food Values of Portions Commonly Used. New York: *Harper & Row, 1989.*

PFEIFFER CC, ET AL. Mental and Elemental Nutrients - A Physician's Guide to Nutrition and Health Care. New Canaan, CT: *Keats Publishing Inc, 1975.*

POSTON C, LISON K. Reclaiming Our Lives. New York: *Little Brown & Co, 1989.*

PRITIKIN N WITH MCGRADY PM JR. The Pritikin Program for Diet and Exercise. New York: *Bantam Books, 1979.*

REMINGTON D, FISHER G, PARENT E. How to Lower Your Fat Thermostat. The No-Diet Reprogramming Plan for Lifelong Weight Control. Provo, Utah: *Vitality House International Inc, 1983.*

RUSH R. The Best Kept Secret. New York: *McGraw-Hill Book Co, 1980.*

SATTILARO AJ WITH MONTE T. Living Well Naturally. Boston: *Houghton Mifflin Co, 1984.*

SCHECHTER SR WITH MONTE T. Fighting Radiation With Foods, Herbs, and Vitamins. Brookline, MA: *East West Health Books, 1988.*

SEIBIN AND TERUKO ARASAKI. "Dietary and medical applications." Vegetables from the Sea. Tokyo: *Japan Publications,1983:32-60.*

SINATRA ST. "Stress management and cardiovascular rehabilitation." The Exercising Adult. Cantu R, ed. New York: *McMillan, 1987.*

STORY JA. "Dietary fiber and lipid metabolism: an update." Medical Aspects of Dietary Fiber. Spiller GA and McP Kay R, eds. p.137. *New York and London: Plenum Medical Books, 1980.*

TARNOWER H, BAKER SS. The Complete Scarsdale Medical Diet plus Dr. Tarnower's Lifetime Keep-Slim Program. New York: *Bantam Books, 1978.*

PERIODICALS

ANDERSON JW, GUSTAFSON NJ, BRYANT CA, TIETYEN-CLARK J. "Dietary fiber and diabetes: a comprehensive review and practical application." J Am Diet Assoc. *1987;87:1189-97.*

ANDERSON JW, ET AL. "Dietary fiber: hyperlipidemia, hypertension, and coronary heart disease." Am J Gastroenterology. *1986;81(10):907-19.*

ANDERSON JW, GUSTAFSON NJ. "High-carohydrate, high-fiber diet. Is it practical and effective in treating hyperlipidemia?" Postgraduate Medicine. *1987;82(4):40.*

AUGUSTI KT, ET AL. "Partial identification of the fibrinolytic activators in onion." Atherosclerosis. *1975;21:409-16.*

BECKER AB, ET AL. "The bronchodilator effects and pharmacolkinetics of caffeine in asthma." NEJM. *March 22, 1984;310(12):743-46.*

BELL LP, HECTOME K, REYNOLDS H, ET AL. "Cholesterol-lowering effects of psyllium hydrophilic nucilloid: adjunct therapy to a prudent diet for patients with mild to moderate hypercholesterolemia." JAMA. *1989;261:3419-23.*

BENFANTE R, REED D. "Is elevated serum cholesterol a risk factor for coronary heart disease in the elderly?" JAMA. *1990;263:393-96.*

BENSON JA JR, ET AL. "Simple chronic constipation." Postgraduate Med. 1975;57:55.

BHASKARAM C, REDDY V. "Cell-mediated immunity in iron- and vitamin-deficient children." BMJ. 1975;3:522.

BLAIR SN, KOHL HW, PAFFENBARGER RS, ET AL. "Physical fitness and all-cause mortality." JAMA. 1989;262:2395-2401.

BLAKE DR, ET AL. "Hypoxic-reperfusion injury in the inflamed human joint." Lancet. 1989 (Feb 11):289-293.

BLANKENHORN DH, KRAMSCH DM. "Reversal of atherosis and sclerosis. The two components of atherosclerosis." Circulation. 1989;79:1-15.

BOHIGIAN MD, PRESENTER. "Dietary fiber and health." Information Report of the Council on Scientific Affairs. AMA. 1988; Apr:1-14.

BORDIA AK. "Effect of garlic on blood lipids in patients with coronary heart disease." Am J Clin Nutr. 1981;34:2100.

BORDIA AK, ET AL. "Essential oil of garlic on blood lipids and fibrinolytic activity in patients with coronary artery disease." Atherosclerosis. 1977;28:155.

BORISH ET, PRIOR WA. "Cigarette smoking, free radicals, and free radical DNA damage. In:Cross CE, moderator, Oxygen radicals and human disease. Ann Int Med. 1987;107:526-545.

BOXER LA, WATANABE AM, ET AL. "Correction of leukocyte function in Chediak-Higashi syndrome by ascorbate." NEJM. 1976;295:1041-45.

BRAY GA. "The energetics of obesity." Twenty-Ninth Annual Meeting of the AC Sports Med. May, 1982.

BROWNLEE S. "Alzheimer's, is there hope?" U.S. News and World Reports. 1991; Aug 12:40-49.

BULRUM RR, CLIFFORD CK, LANZA E. "NCI dietary guidelines: rationale." Am J Clin Nutr. 1988;48:888-95.

BURKITT DP, WALKER ARP, PAINTER NS. "Dietary fiber and disease." JAMA. 1974;229:1068.

BURKITT DP. "Some disease characteristic of modern western civilization." BMJ. 1973;1:274.

BURTON GW, INGOLD KU. "Beta-carotene: an unusual type of lipid antioxidant." Science. 1984;224:569-573.

CAMAIONE DN, SINATRA ST. "Beneficial effects of exercise and current concepts in adult fitness." CT Med. *1981;45(10):620-25.*

CHIHARA G, ET AL. "Fractionation and purification of the polysacchrides with marked antitumor activity, especially lentinan, from LENTINUS EDODES (Berk.)Sing.(an edible mushroom)." Cancer Res. *30,1970;2776-81.*

COOPER KH. "Coronary combat." Modern Maturity. *Dec 1988-Jan 1989:78-84.*

CLEARY-MERKER L. "Childhood sexual abuse as an antecedent to obesity." The Bariatrician, AM J Bariatric Med. *Spring, 1991;17-22.*

COSTILL DL, ET AL. "Effects of caffeine ingestion on metabolism and exercise performance." Medicine and Science in Sports. *1978;10(3):155-58.*

COX IM. "Magnesium Therapy Improves Symptoms of Chronic Fatigue Syndrome." Lancet. *Southampton, UK;1991,337:757-60.*

CUMMINGS JH, ET AL. "Colonic response to dietary fiber from carrot, cabbage, apple, bran and guar gum." Lancet. *January 7, 1978;5-8.*

D'AGOSTINO RB, BELANGER AJ, KANNEL WB. "Relations of Low Diastolic Blood Pressure to Coronary Heart Disease Death in Presence of Myocardial Infarction: the Framingham Study." BMJ. *August 17, 1991;303:385-89.*

DYCKNER T, WESTER PO. "Potassium/magnesium depletion in patients with cardiovascular disease." Am J of Med. *March 1987;62:11-17.*

FACCHINETTI F, BORELLA P, SANCES G, ET AL. "Oral magnesium successfully relieves premenstrual mood changes." Obstetrics & Gynecology. *August 1991;78:2:177-81.*

"Fish Oil." The Medical Letter. *January 11, 1991:4.*

FOSTER WR, BURTON BT. "Health implications of obesity." Ann Int Med. *1985;103:1024-30.*

FRAMBACH DA AND RICK EB. Letter to the editor regarding "Zinc supplementation and anemia." JAMA. *February 20, 1991;265(7):879.*

GILES TD. "Magnesium deficiency: an important cardiovascular risk factor." Advances in Cardiology. *1990;1(5).*

GILES TD, CHOBANIAN MD. "Magnesium deficiency: a new cardiovascular risk factor in sudden cardiac death." A Symposium. *1990.*

"Girth and Death." Metropolitan Life Ins Co. *1939.*

GLOTH FM III, ET AL. "Can vitamin D deficiency produce an unusual pain syndrome?" Arch Intern Med. *August 1991;151:1662-64.*

GOLDSMITH M. "Will exercise keep women away from oncologists or obstetricians?" JAMA. *1988;259(12):1769-70.*

GOTTO AM JR chairman. "Atherosclerosis, a decade in perspective." Highlights of symposium sponsored by Baylor College of Medicine. *Winter 1991.*

GREENBERG SM, FRISHMAN WH. "Coenzyme Q10: A new drug for myocardial ischemia?" The Medical Clinics of North America. *1988;72(1):243-258.*

GREENBERG SM, FRISHMAN WH. "Co-enzyme Q10: A new drug for cardiovascular disease." Journal of Clinical Pharmacology. *1990;30:596-608.*

GREISER EM, MASCHEWSKI-SCHNEIDER U, TEMPEL G, HELMERT U. "Smoking, medication found to increase cholesterol levels." Cardiology World News. *1991; Sept:26-27.*

GRUNDY SM. "Cholesterol and coronary heart disease, future directions." JAMA. *1990;264(23):3053-59.*

GRUNDY SM. "Comparison of monounsaturated fatty acids and carbohydrates for lowering plasma cholesterol." NEJM. *March 20, 1986;314(12):745-48.*

GRUNDY SM. "High serum cholesterol: treatment by diet." Cardiology Board Review. *1989;6(3):32-8.*

HABER JB, HEATON KW, MURPHY D, BURROUGHS LF. "Depletion and disruption of dietary fiber: effect on satiety, plasma, glucose and serum insulin." Lancet. *1977;2:679.*

HARMAN D. "Free radicals: aging and disease." In:Cross CE, moderator, Oxygen radicals and human disease. Ann Int Med. *1987;526-545.*

"Harvard Heart Letter." Harvard Medical School. *1991;2(1):1-7.*

HENNEKENS CH. Personal communication at Hartford Cardiovascular Symposium. *1991.*

HENNEKENS CH, ET AL. "Final report on the aspirin component of the ongoing physicians' health study." NEJM. *1989;321:129-35.*

HEROLD KC AND HEROLD BC. Letter to the editor regarding "Benefits and risks of exercise." JAMA. *June 3, 1983;249:21.*

HUAG A. Composition and Properties of Alginates, Report No. 30. Trondheim: Norw Seaweed Res Inst, *1964.*

JACKSON R, SCRAGG R, BEAGLEHOLE R. "Alcohol Consumption and risk of coronary heart disease." BMJ. *1991;303:211.*

JAIN RC, ET AL. "Onion and blood fibrinolytic activity." BMJ. *1969;258:514.*

KAMIKAWA T, KOBAYASHI A, YAMASHITA T, ET AL. "Effects of coenzyme Q10 on exercise tolerance in chronic stable angina pectoria." Am J Card. *1985;56(4):247-251.*

KAPLAN JR, MANUCK SB, CLARKSON TB, ET AL. "Social status, environment, and atherosclerosis in cynomolgus monkeys." Arteriosclerosis. *1982;2(5):359-68.*

KEYS A, ET AL. "The diet and 15-year death rate in the seven countries study." Am J Epid. *December 1986;124(6):903-15.*

KOK FJ, MARTIN RF, MERVYN L, ET AL. "Selenium, cancer foe." Better Nutrition for Today's Living. *November, 1990*

KOPLAN JP, POWELL KE, SILKES RK, ET AL. "An epidemiological study of the benefits and risks of running." JAMA *1982;248(23):3118-21.*

KIRBY RW, ET AL. "Oat-bran intake selectively lowers serum low-density lipoprotein cholesterol concentrations of hypercholesterolemic men." Am J Clin Nutr. *May 1981;34:824-29.*

LANZA E, JONES Y, BLOCK G, KESSLER L. "Dietary fiber intake in the US population." Am J Clin Nutr. *1987;46:790-97.*

LAU BHS, ET AL. "Allium sativum (garlic) and atherosclerosis: a review." Nutr Res. *1983;3:119-28.*

LAUER MS, ANDERSON KM, KANNEL WB, ET AL. "The impact of obesity on left ventricular mass and geometry. The Framingham heart study." JAMA. *July 10, 1991;266(2):231-36.*

LEAF A, WEBER PC. "Cardiovascular effects of n-3 fatty acids: an update." NEJM. *1988;318:549-57.*

MACNEIL LEHRER REPORT. "Eat smart." *September 16, 1991.*

MARX JL. "Oxygen free radicals linked to many diseases." Science. *1987;235:529-531.*

MAUER I, BERNHARD A, ZIERZ S. "Coenzyme Q10 and respiratory chain enzyme activities in hypertrophied human left ventricles with aortic valve stenosis." Am J of Cardiology. *August 15, 1990;66:504-05.*

McBarron J. "Bariatrics." The Bariatrician, Am J Bariatric Med. *Spring, 1991:9-16.*

McCord JM. "Oxygen-derived free radicals in postischemic tissue injury." NEJM. *1985;312(3):159-163.*

Metropolitan Life Insurance Company: 1983 Metropolitan Height and Weight Table. Reprinted courtesy of Metropolitan Life Insurance Company.

Metz R. "Obesity: an eclectic review." Hosp Pract. *1987;22(2)152.*

Millane TA, Ward De, Camm AJ, "Is hypomagnesemia arrhythmogenic?" Clinical Cardiology. *1992;15:103-108.*

Morris JN, Heady JA, Raffle PAB, et al. "Coronary heart disease and physical activity of work." Lancet. *1953;2:1053.*

Morris JN, Kogan A, Patterson DC, et al. "Incidence and prediction of ischemic heart disease in London busmen." Lancet. *1966;2:553.*

"Multiple risk factor intervention trial." JAMA. *1982;248:1465-77.*

National Heart, Lung, and Blood Institute, National Institute of Health, US Department of Health and Human Services. "National cholesterol education program, report of the expert panel in population strategies for blood cholesterol reduction: executive summary." Arch of Int Med. *June, 1991;151:1071-84.*

Nerem RM, Levesque MJ, Cornhill JF, et al. "Social environment as a factor in diet-induced atherosclerosis." Science. *1980;208:1475.*

"Nutritional Trends." Internal Medicine News. *1991; July 15-31:30.*

Ornish D, et al. "Can lifestyle changes reverse coronary heart disease? The lifestyle heart trial." Lancet. *1990;336:129-33.*

"Pectin may reduce cholesterol, colon cancer incidence." Cardiology World News. *1991; Sept:8.*

Prescott L. "Symposium: magnesium in clinical medicine and therapeutics. Wide range of diseases linked to low magnesium levels."

Intrn Med World Rpt. *June 15,30, 1991:7.*

Pomare EW, Heaton KW. "Alteration of bile salt metabolism by dietary fiber (bran)." BMJ. *1973;4:262.*

Psyllium and rice bran: more obscure than oat bran – but they lower cholesterol, too." Mayo Clin Nutr Lett. *1990;3(7):1-2.*

221

Ravussin E, Lillioja S, Knowler WC, et al. "Reduced rate of energy expenditure as a risk factor for body-weight gain." NEJM. *1988;318:467-72.*

Riemersma RA, Wood DA, MacIntyre CC, et al. Abstract:"Risk of angina rises with low vitamin E, C, and carotene intake." Modern Medicine. *1991;59:68.*

Roberts SB, Savage J, Coward WA, et al. "Energy expenditure and intake in infants born to lean and overweight mothers." NEJM. *1988;318:461-66.*

Roubenoff, RA. "Nutritional risk factors in cardiovascular disease, part 18 Omega-3 fatty acids and coronary heart disease." Choices in Cardiology. *1990;4(6):297-98.*

Roubenoff RA. "Nutritional risk factors in cardiovascular disease, part 21, Maintaining adequate calcium intake on low-fat diets." Choices in Cardiology. *1991.*

Roubenoff RA. "Nutritional risk factors in cardiovascular disease, part 22, Dietary guidelines for healthy American adults." Choices in Cardiology. *1991;5(4):165-66.*

Sheffy BE, Schultz RD. "Influence of vitamin E and selenium on immune response mechanisms." Fed Proc. *1979;38:2139-43.*

Shirlow MJ, et al. "A study of caffeine consumption and symptoms; indigestion, palpitations, tremor, headache and insomnia." Int J Epid. *June 1985;14(2):239-48.*

Siegel AJ. "New insights about obesity and exercise." Your Patient and Fitness. *1988;2(6):6-13.*

Sinatra ST. "Stress - a cardiologists point of view." Postgraduate Med. *1984;76:231-34.*

Sinatra ST. "Stress and the heart - behavioral interaction and plan for strategy." CT Med. *1984;48:81-86.*

Sinatra ST, et al. "Effects of continuous passive motion, walking, and a placebo intervention on physical and psychological well-being." J Cardiopul Rehab. *August 1990;10(8)279-86.*

Sinatra ST, Chawla S. "Aortic dissection associated with anger, suppressed rage, and cute emotional stress." J Cardiopul Rehab. *1986;6(5).*

Sinatra ST, Feitell LA. "The heart and mental stress, real and imagined." Lancet. *1985; 223-223.*

Sirtori CR, et al. "Controlled evaluation of fat intake in the Mediterranean diet: comparative activities of olive oil and corn oil on plasma lipids and platelets in high-risk patients." Am J Clin Nutr. *1986;44:635-42.*

Sismann G, et al. ILIB Advisory Board. "Focus on diet and exercise." Lipid Digest. *1988; 1(2):1-6.*

Snider, Mike. "Doctors Urge Lowering Dietary Fat to 25%." USA Today. *1991.*

Southorn PA. "Free radicals in medicine. 1. Chemical nature and biologic reactions." Mayo Clin Proc. *1988;63:381-389.*

Spiller GA, Gates JE. "Effect of Diets High in Monounsaturated Fats, Plant Proteins and Complex Carbohydrates on Serum Lipoproteins in Hypercholesterolemic Humans." Internation Symposium on Drugs Affecting Lipid Metabolism. *Nov 8-11, 1989.*

Steen SN, Oppliger RA, Brownell KD. "Metabolic effects of repeated weight loss and regain in adolescent wrestlers." JAMA. *1988;260(1):47-50.*

Swain JF, Rouse IL, Curley CB, Sacks FM. "Comparison of the effects of oat bran and low-fiber wheat on serum lipoprotein levels and blood pressure." NEJM. *1990;322:147-52.*

Subak-Sharpe GJ, Hammock DA, "The Family Circle Pocket Nutrition Counter." Family Circle Magazine. *1991.*

Tanaka J, Tominaga R, Yoshitoshi M, et al. "Coenzyme Q10: "The prophylactic effect on low cardiac output following cardiac valve replacement." The Annals of Thoracic Surgery. *1982;33:145-151.*

Tappel A. "Vitamin E spares the parts of the cell and tissues from free radical damage." Nutrition Today. *1973;8:4.*

Teas J. "The consumption of seaweed as a protective factor in the etiology of breast cancer." Med Hypotheses. *1981;7:(5)601-13.*

Thompson PD, Funk EJ, Carleton RA, et al. "Incidence of death during jogging in Rhode Island from 1975-1980." JAMA. *1982;247(18):2535-38.*

"Twelve weeks to a healthier diet." Choices in Cardiology. *1991;5(4):167-68.*

Vallance S. "Relationship between ascorbic acid and serum proteins of the immune system." BMJ. *1977;2:437-38.*

VanCamp SP. "The Hazards of exercise." Your Patient and Fitness. *1987;1(4):18-21.*

WALKER ARP, BURKITT DP. "Colonic cancer: hypotheses of causation, dietary prophylaxis and future research." Am J Clin Nutr. *1976(1978)31:910.*

WEINER MA. "Cholesterol in foods rich in omega-3 fatty acids." NEJM. *1986;315:833.*

WEISBURGER, JH. "Nutritional approach to cancer prevention with emphasis on vitamins, antioxidants, and carotenoids." Am J Clin Nutr. *1991;53:226S-37S.*

WHANG R. "Magnesium deficiency: Pathogenesis, prevalence, and clinical implications." Am J of Med. *March 20, 1987;82:24-29.*

WILBER, JF. "Neuropeptides, appetite regulation, and human obesity." JAMA. *1991;266(2):257-58.*

WYNDER EL, SHIGEMATSU T. "Environmental factors of cancer of the colon and rectum." Cancer. *1967;20:1520.*

INDEX